PICTURE BOOK OF
FLOWERS

"Many eyes go through the meadow,
but few see the flowers in it."
- Ralph Waldo Emerson

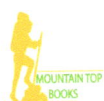

Copyright © 2023 Mountain Top Books
www.amazon.com/author/mountaintopbooks
All Rights Reserved.

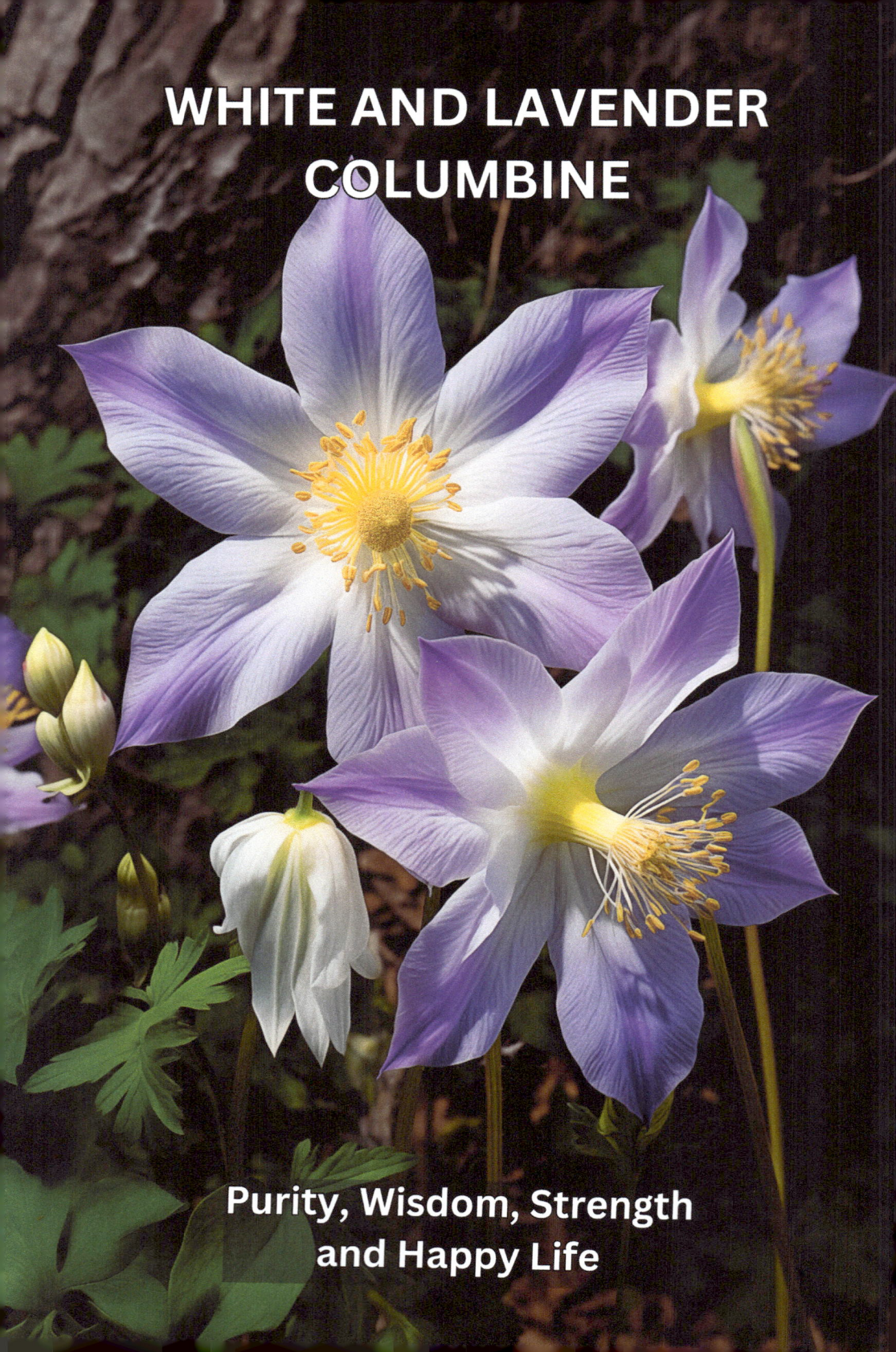

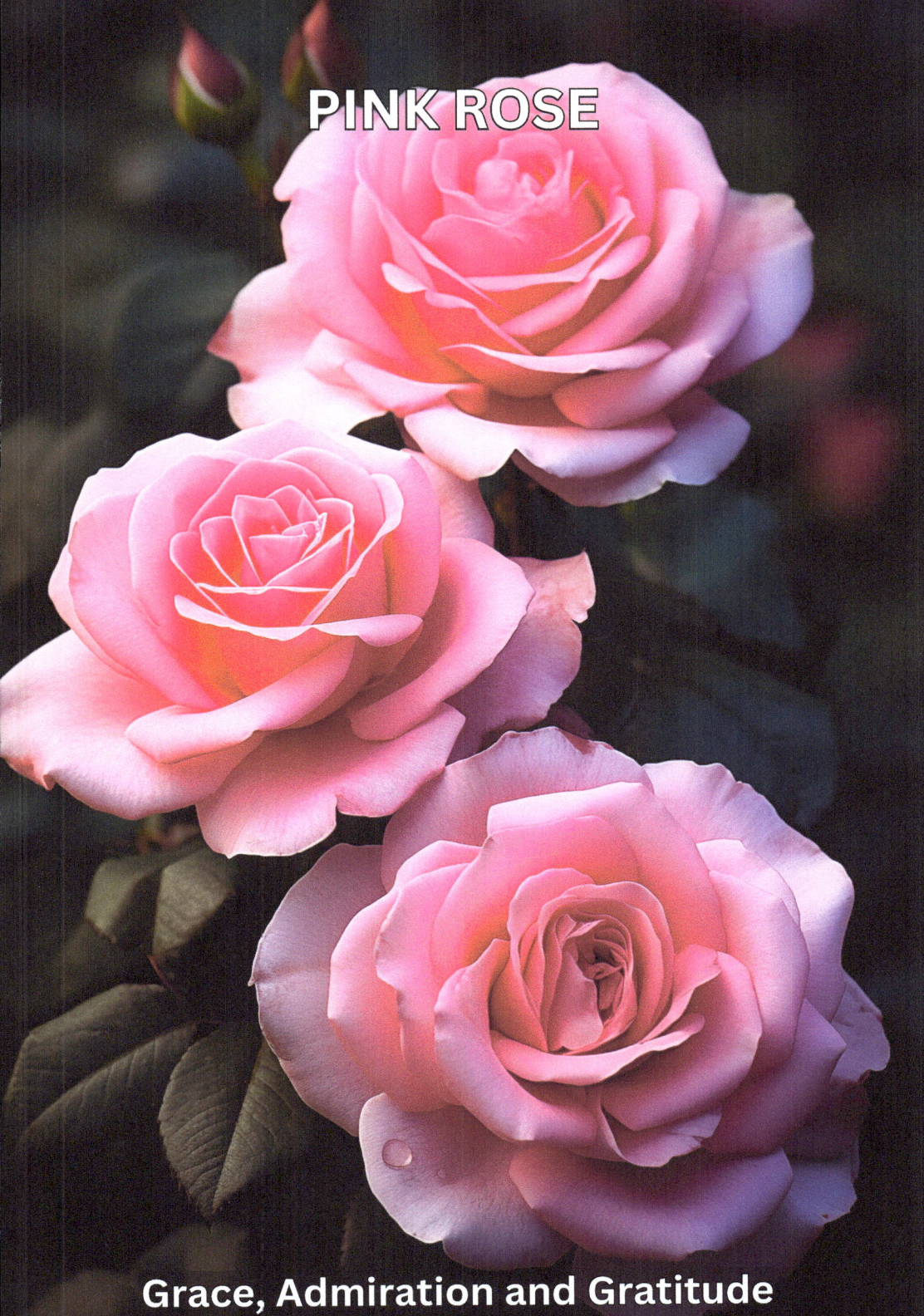

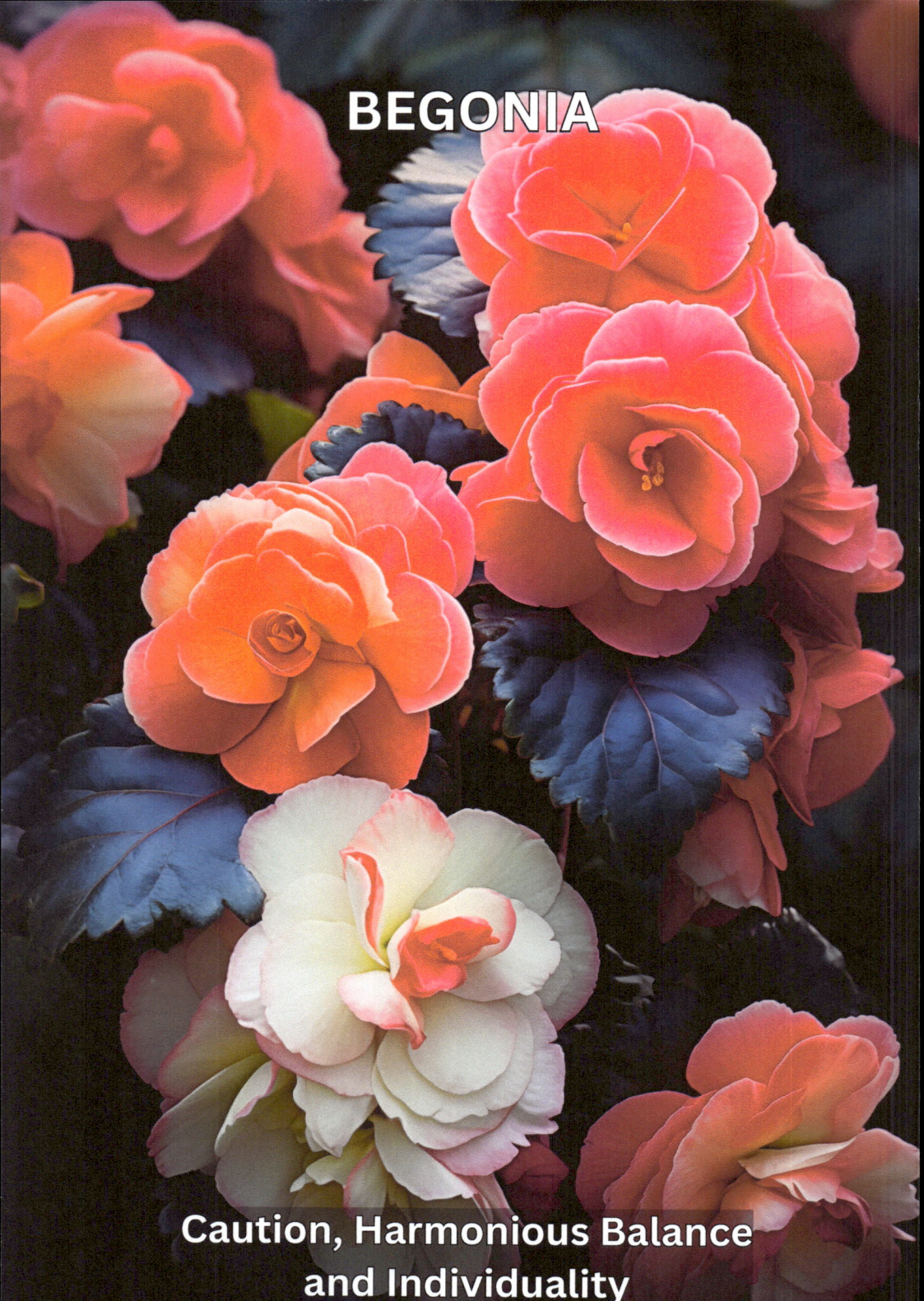

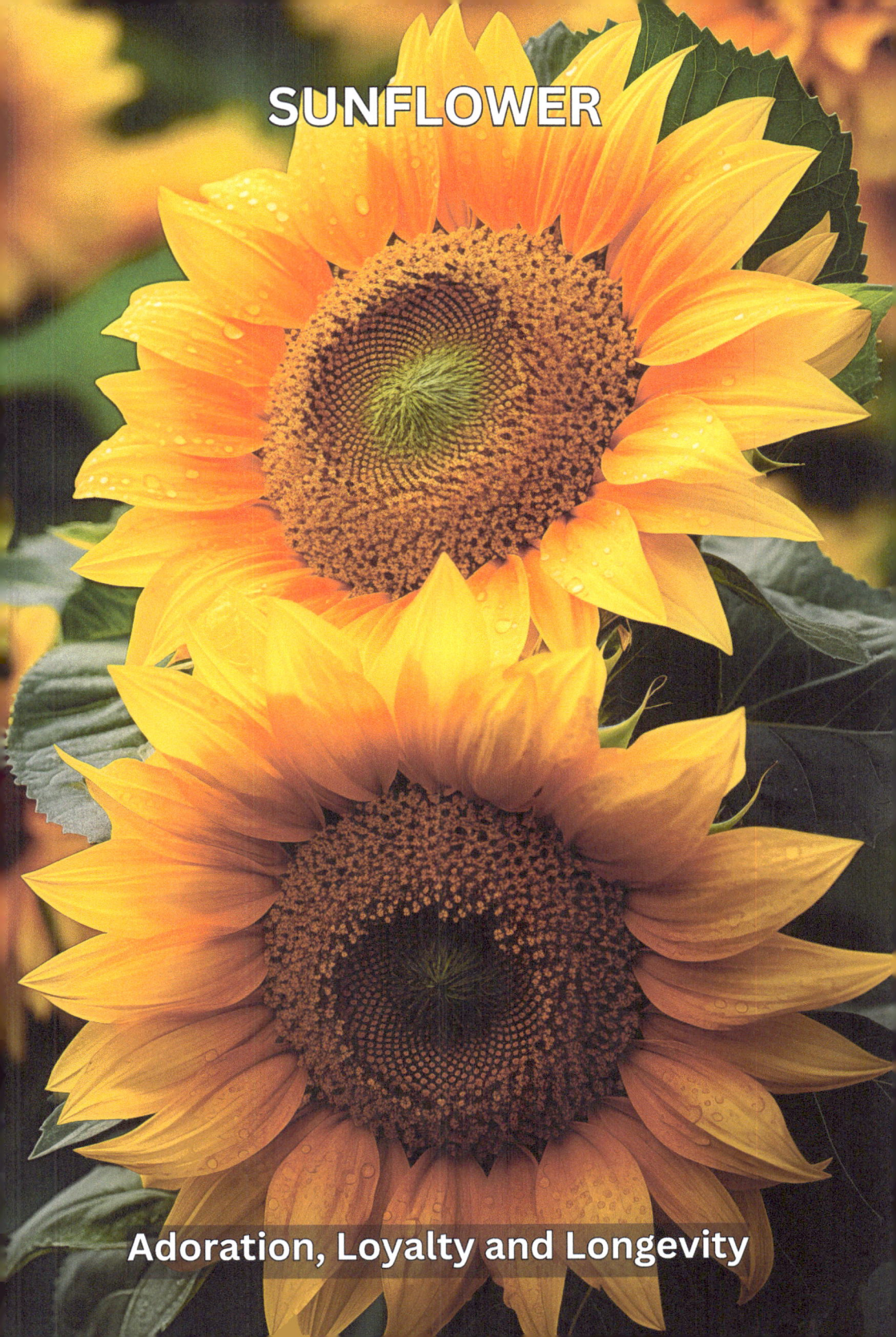

CARNATION

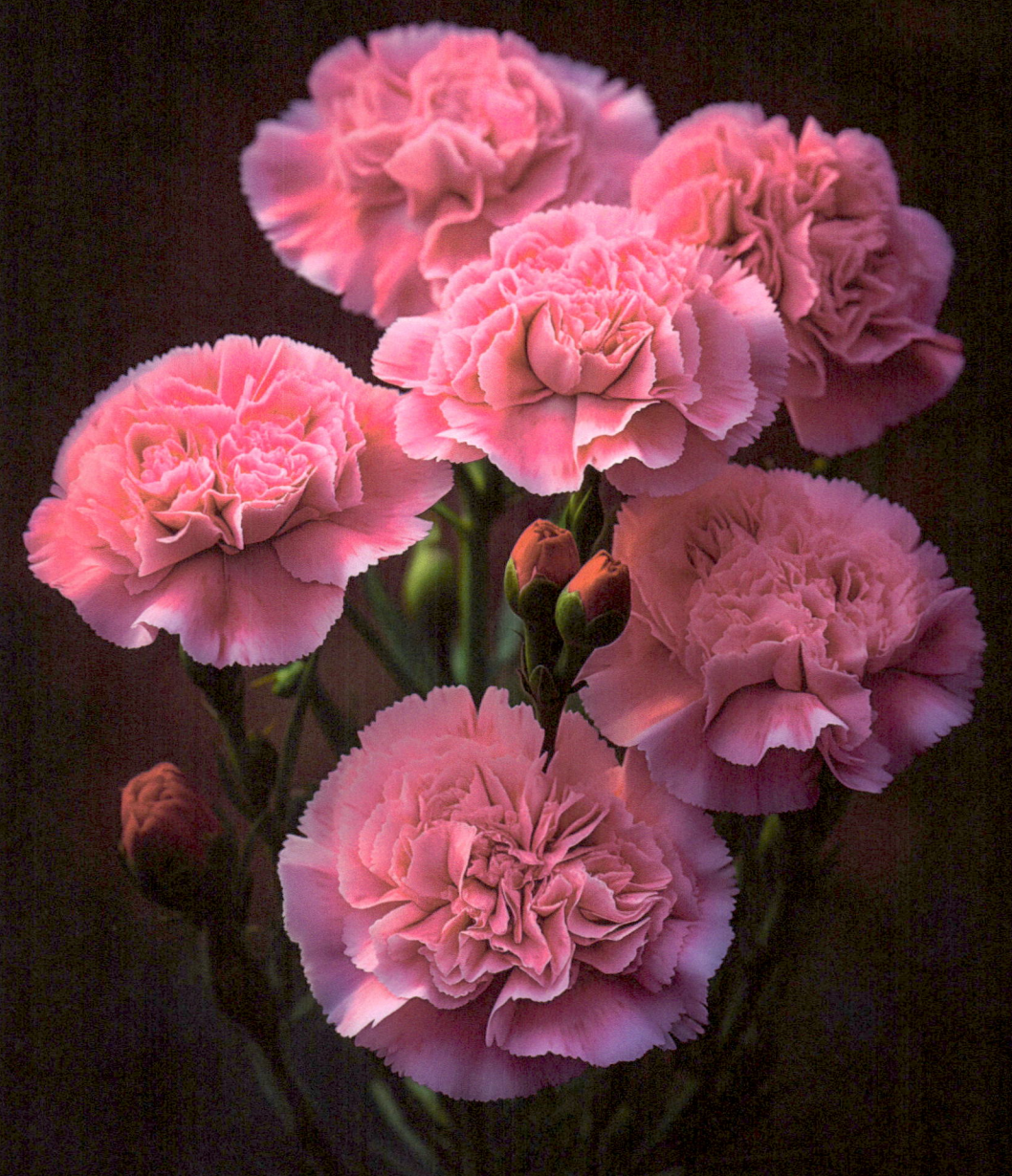

Love, Fascination and Distinction

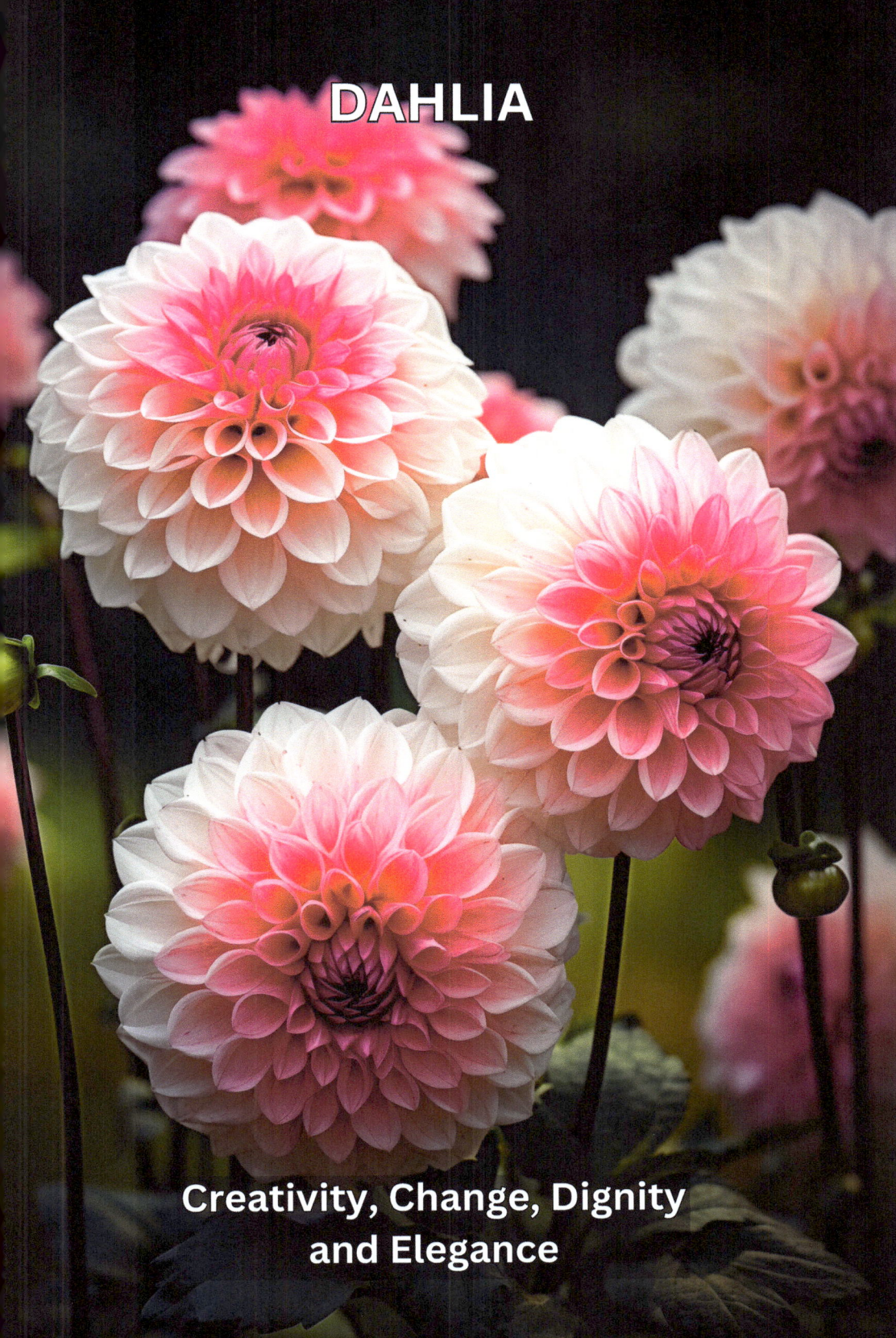

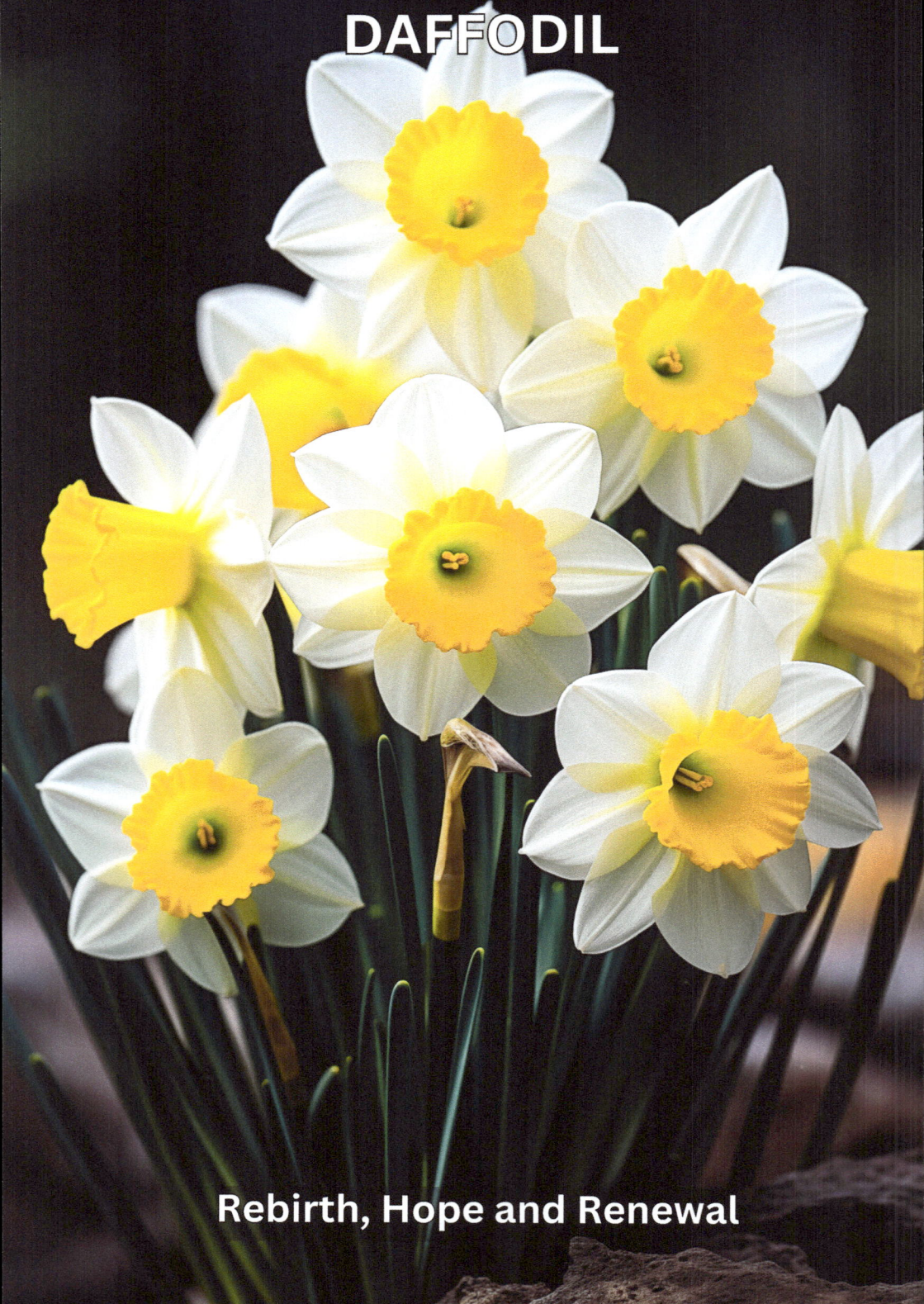

GERBERA DAISY

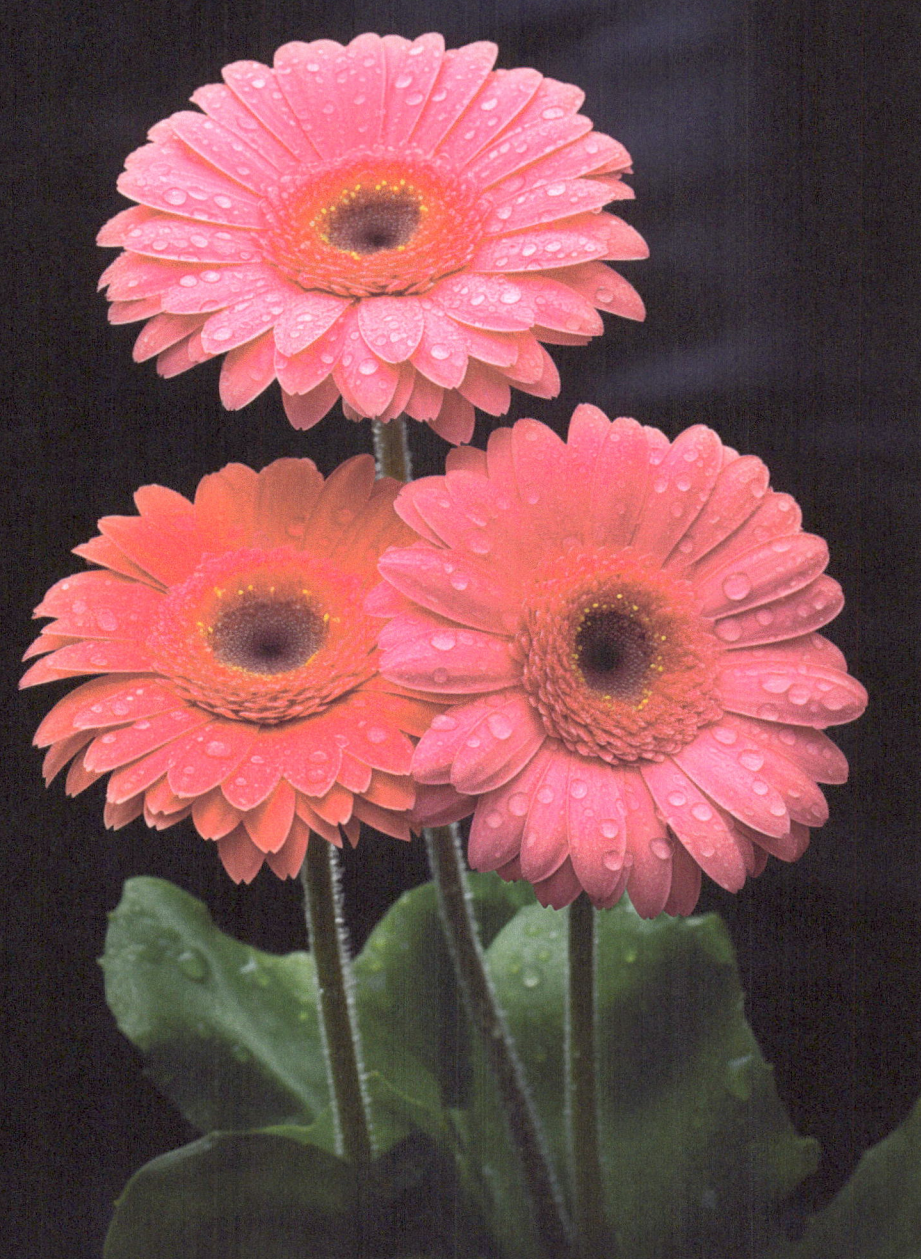

Beauty, Joy and Purity

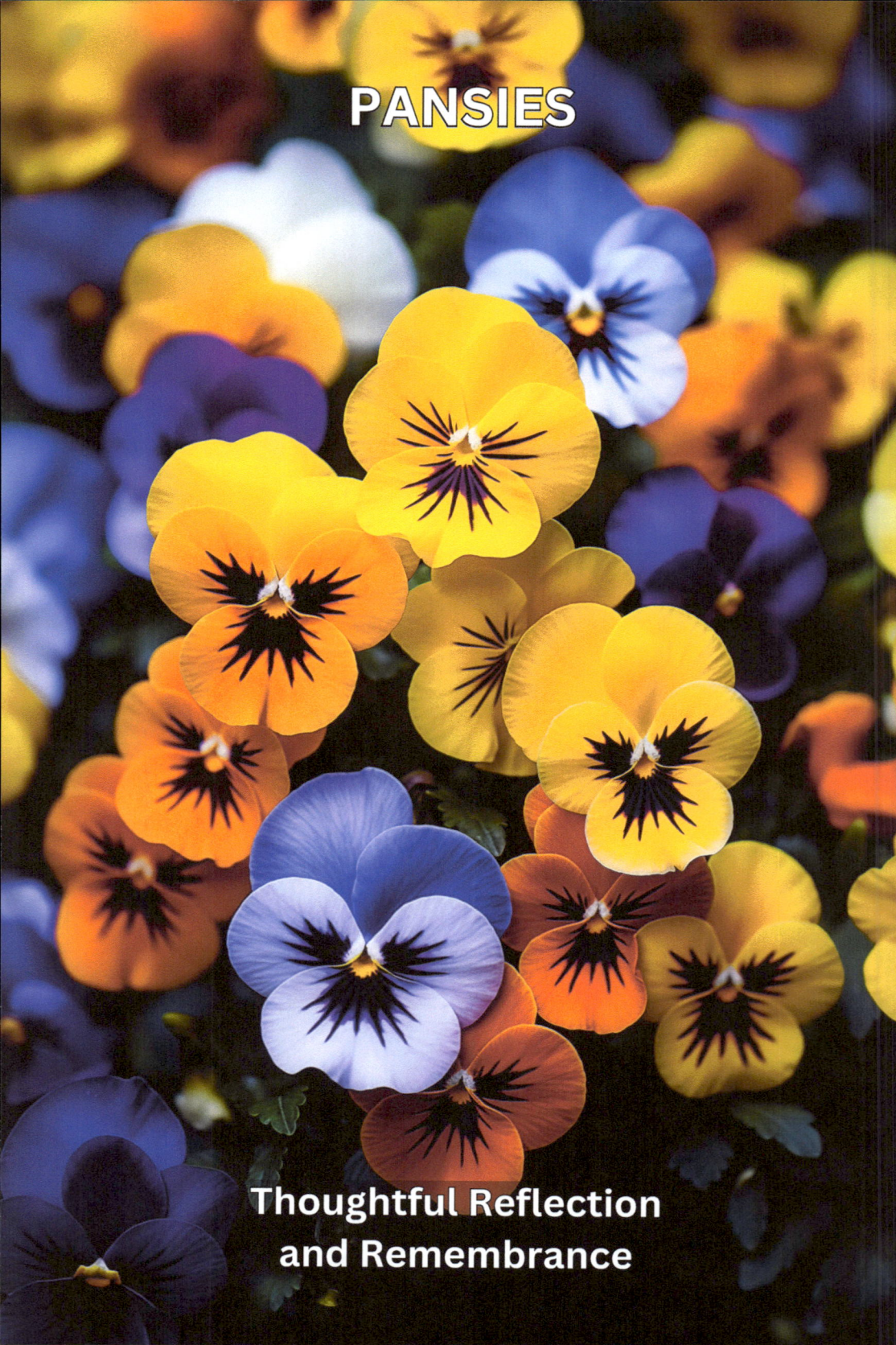

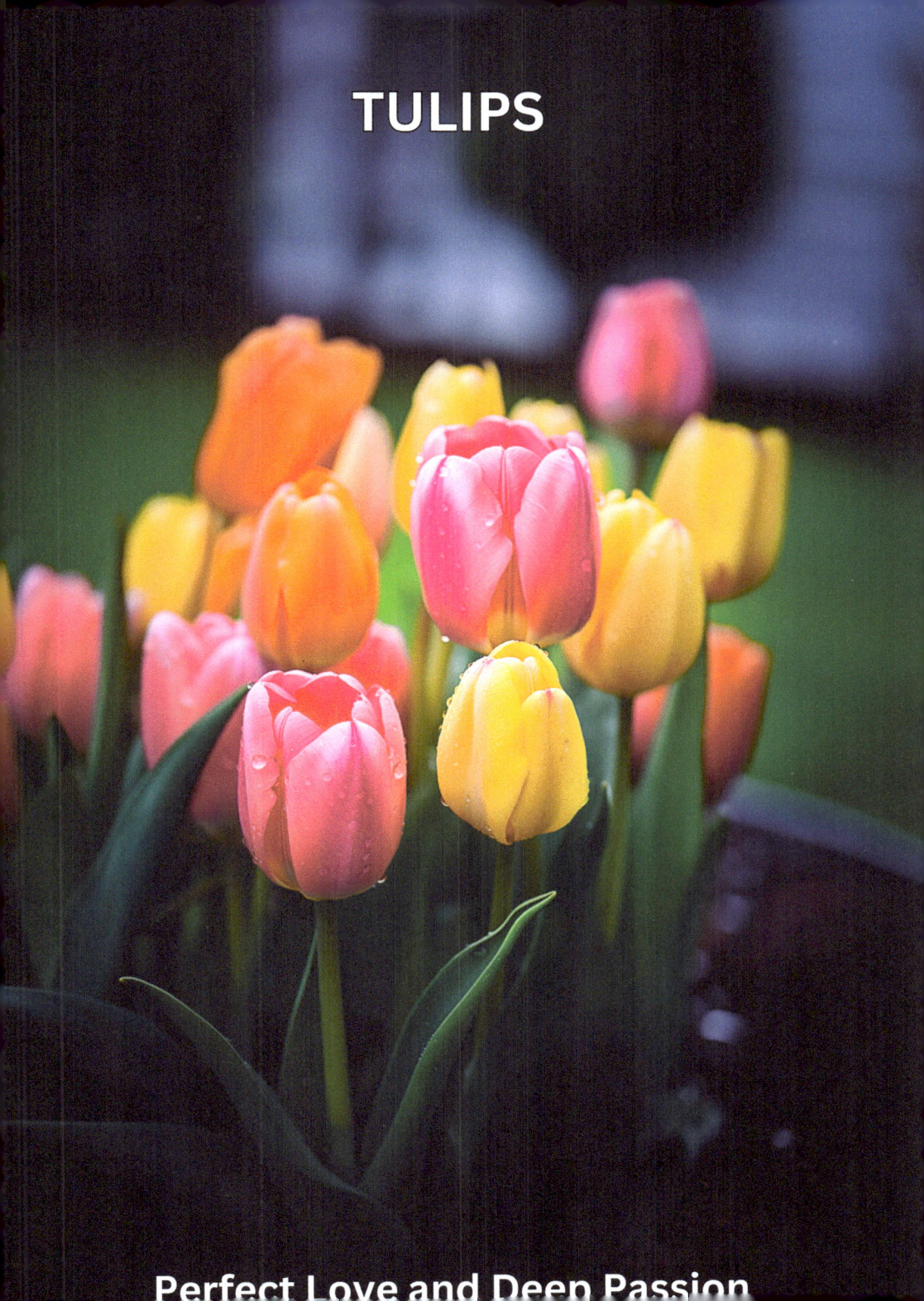
TULIPS

Perfect Love and Deep Passion

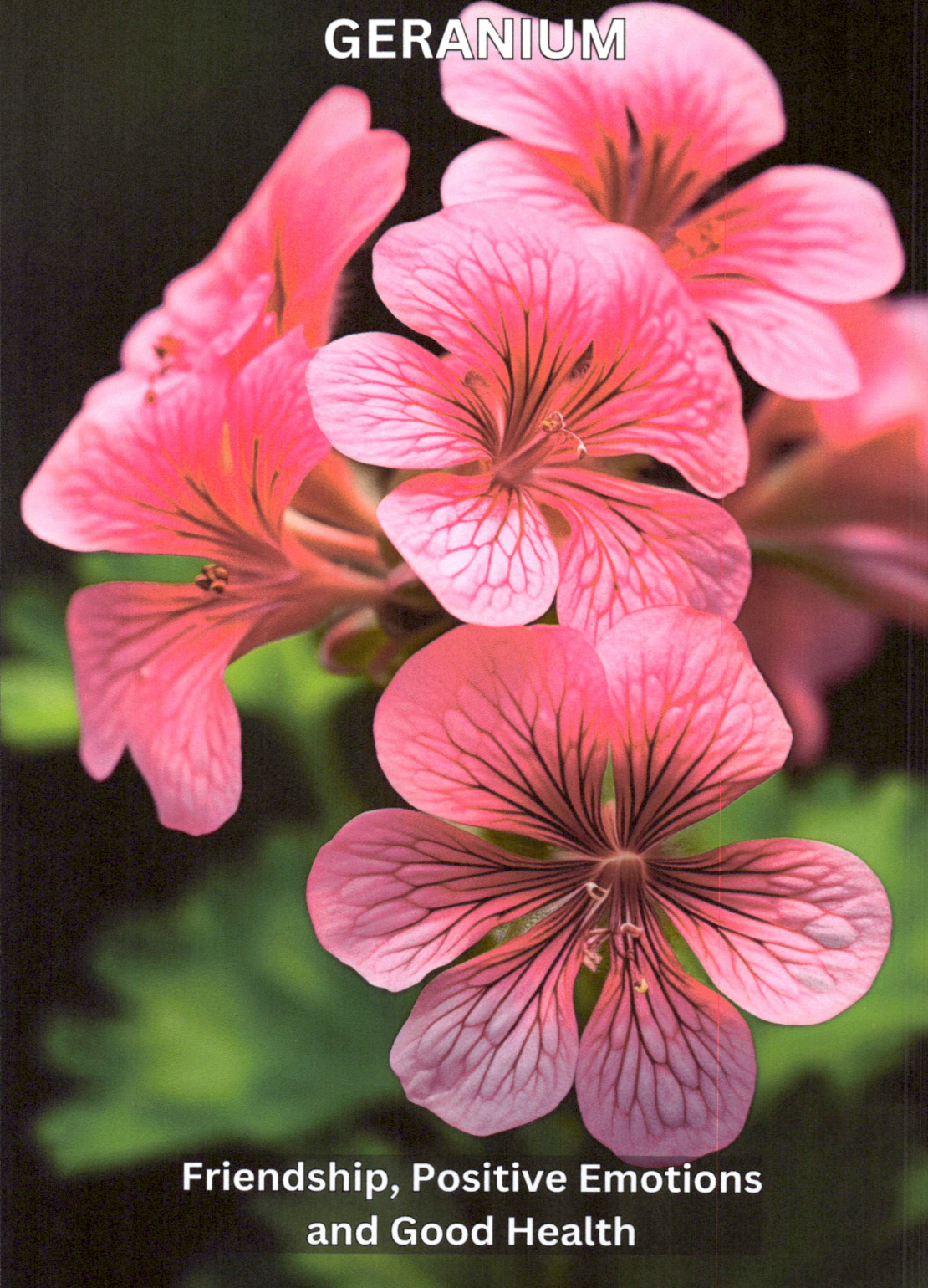

GERANIUM

Friendship, Positive Emotions and Good Health

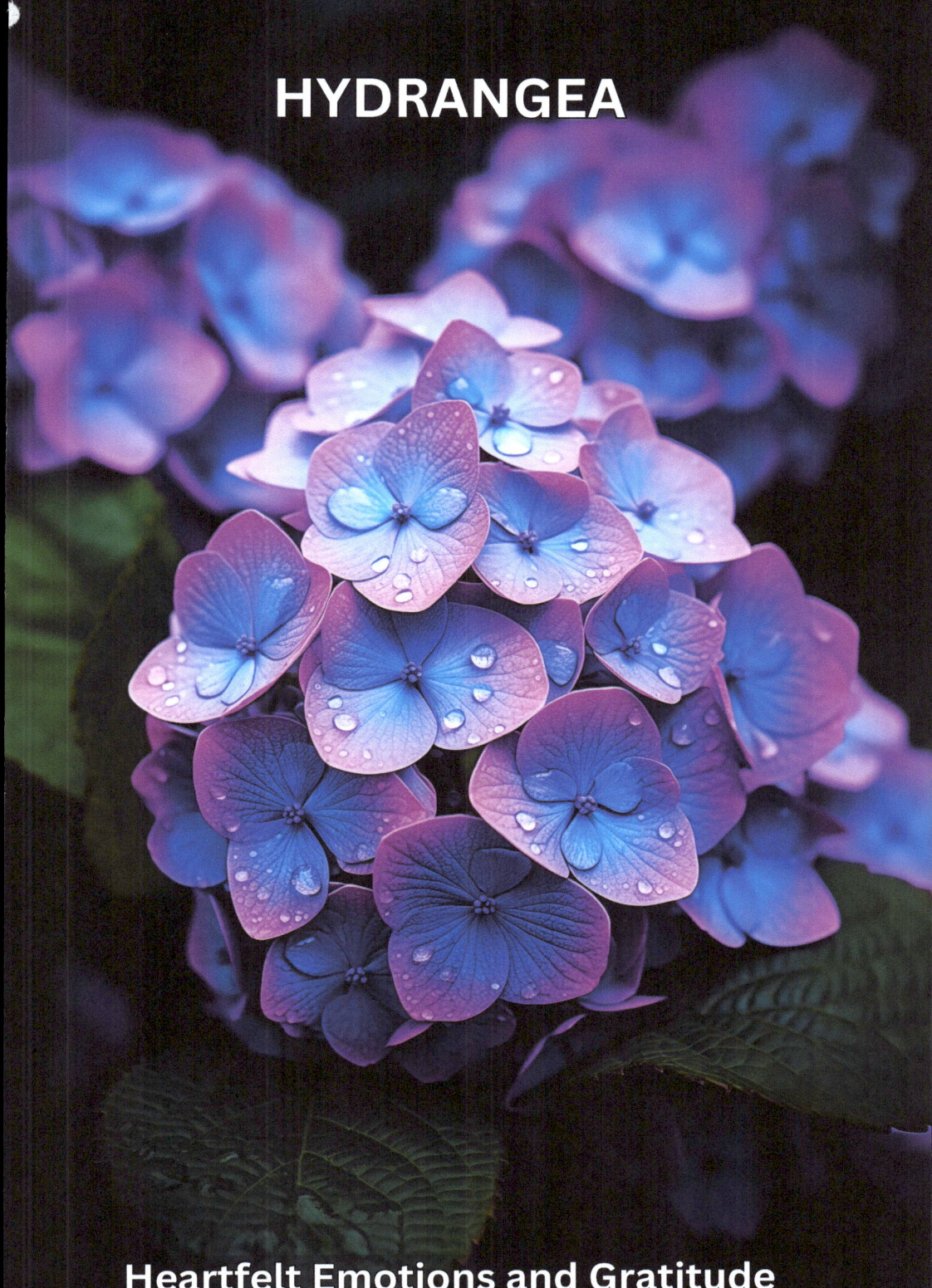

GLADIOLI

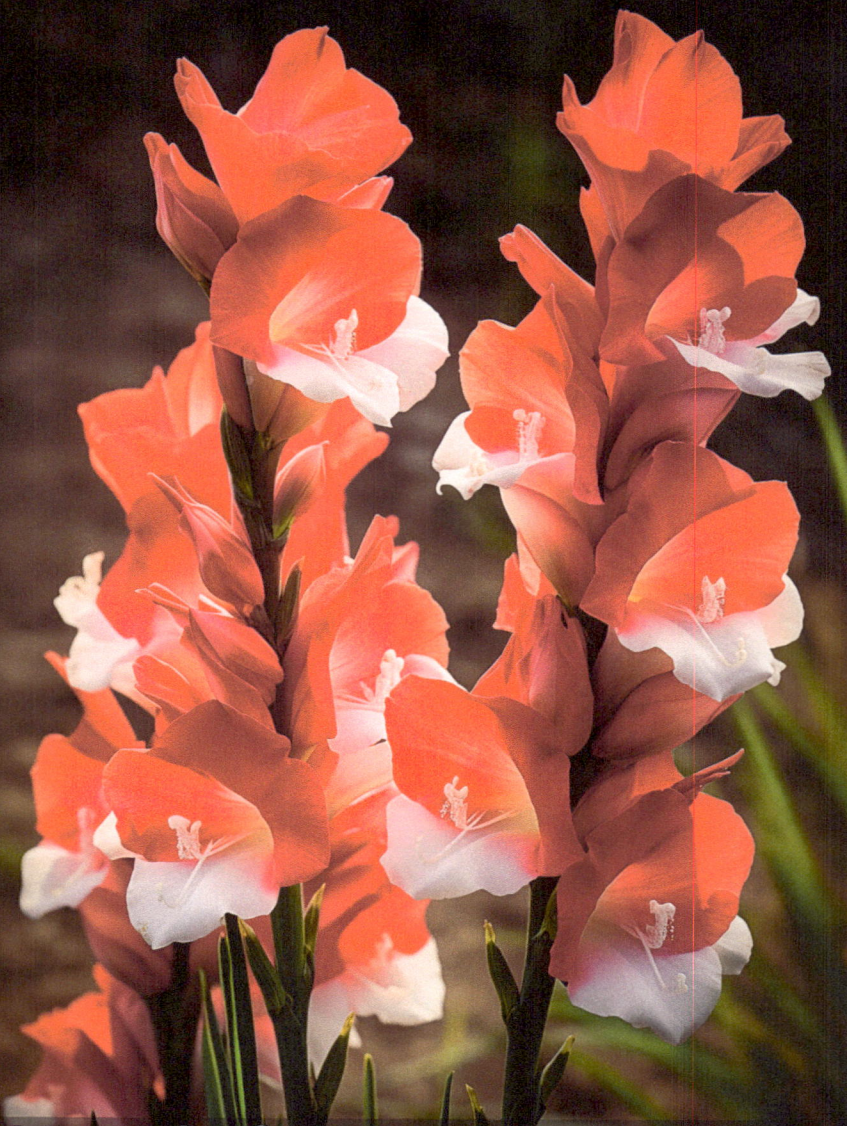

Strength of Character, Faithfulness and Honor
Name Comes From the Latin Word "Gladius," for Sword

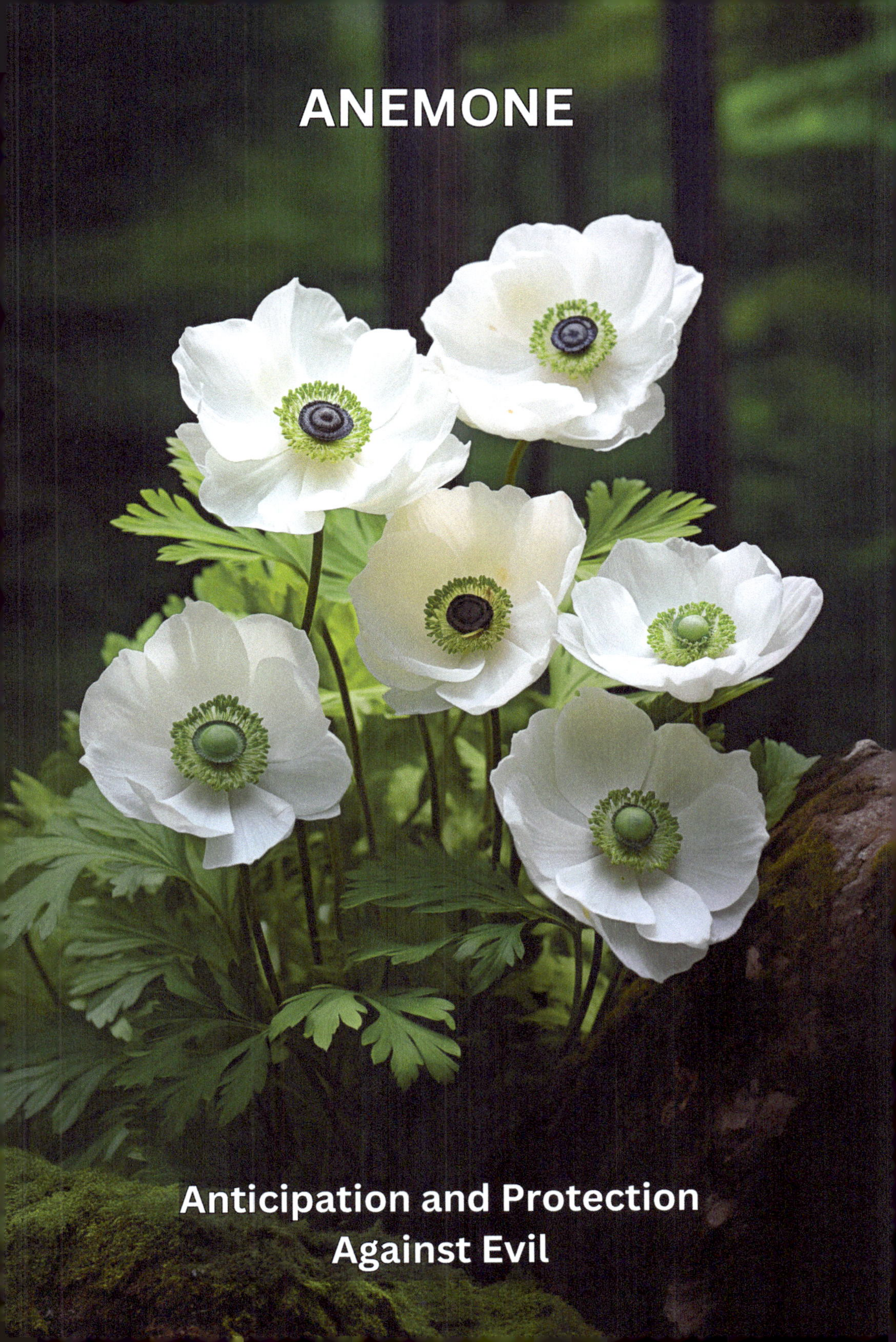

ANEMONE

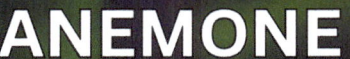

Anticipation and Protection Against Evil

IRIS

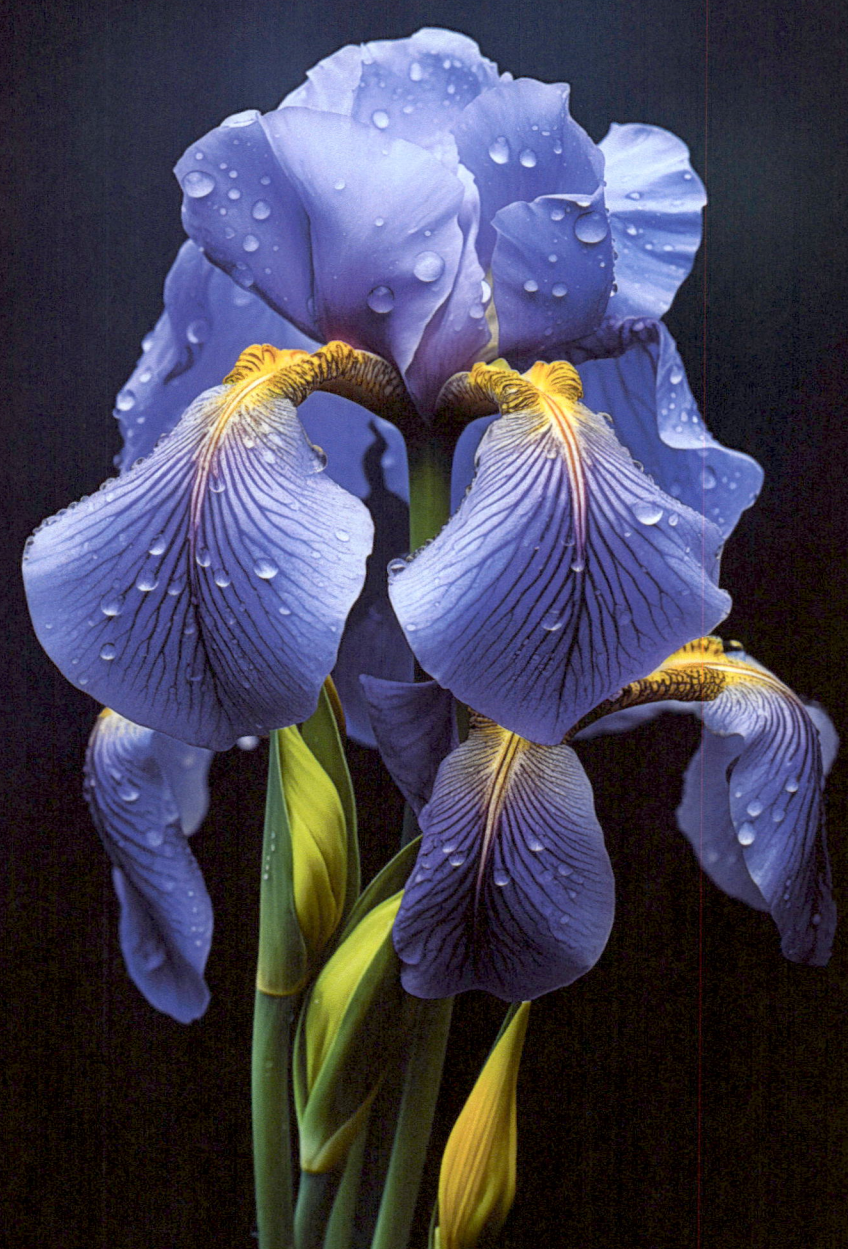

Royalty, Valor, Wisdom, Hope and Trust

CHRYSANTHEMUMS

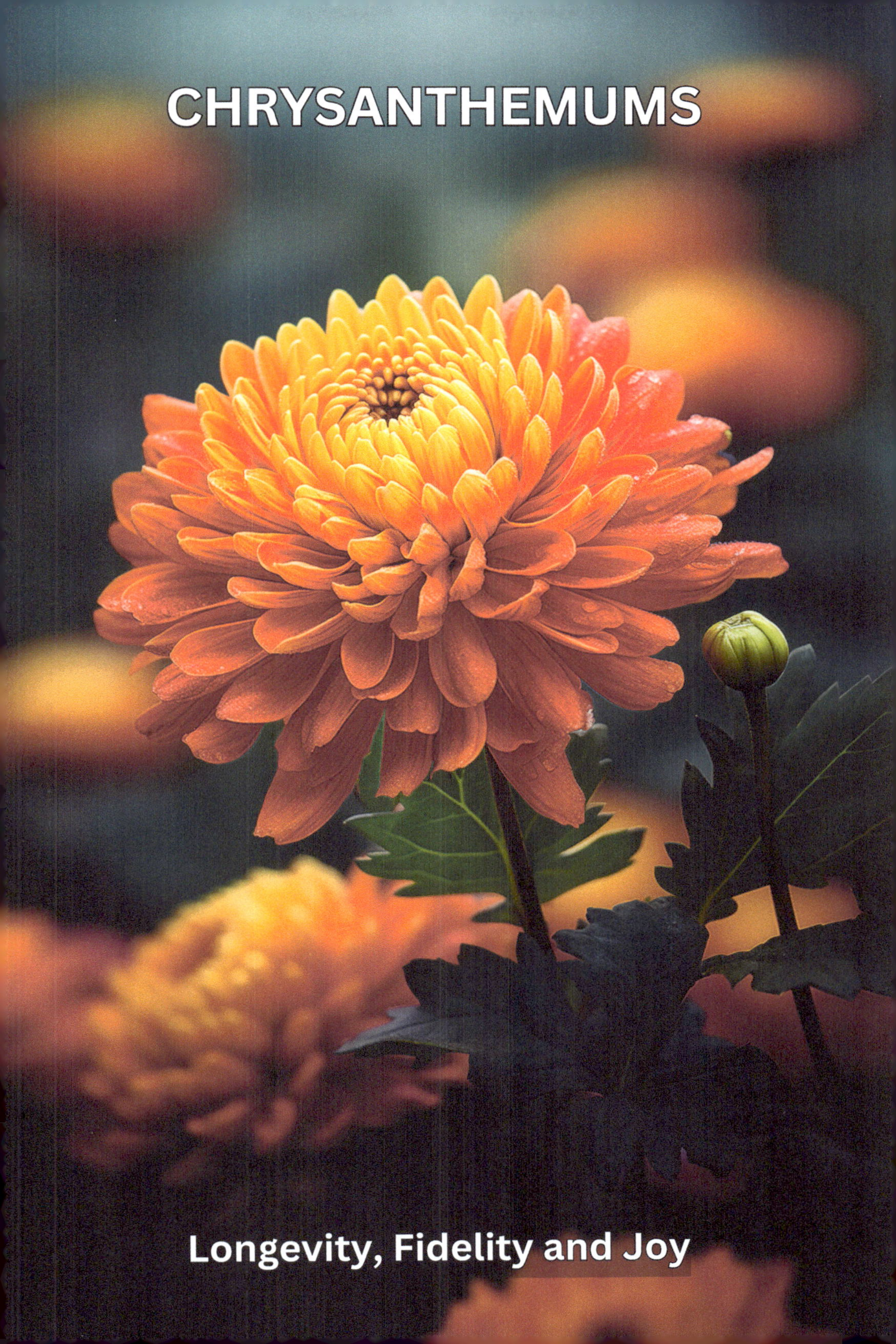

Longevity, Fidelity and Joy

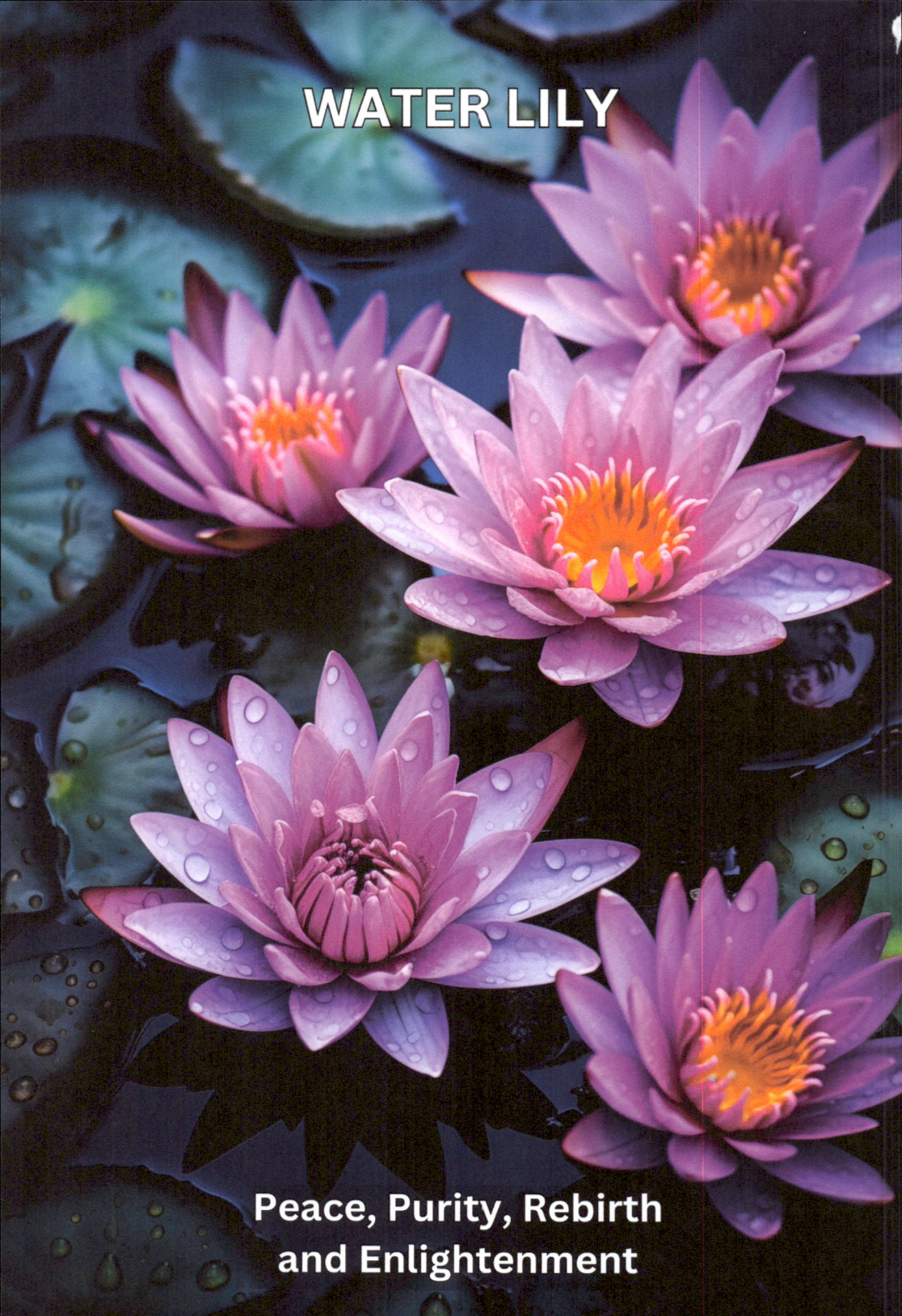

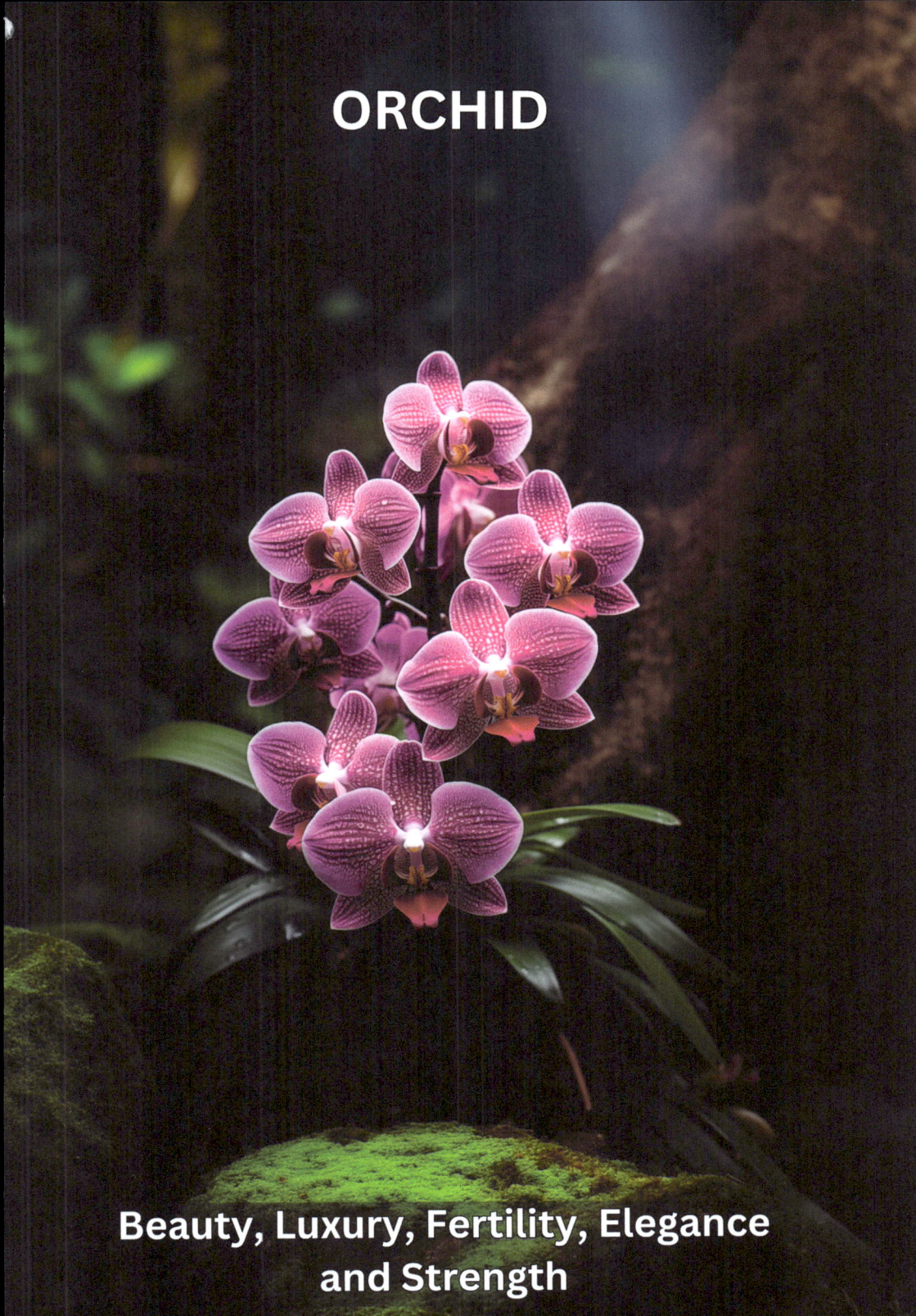

FORGET-ME-NOT

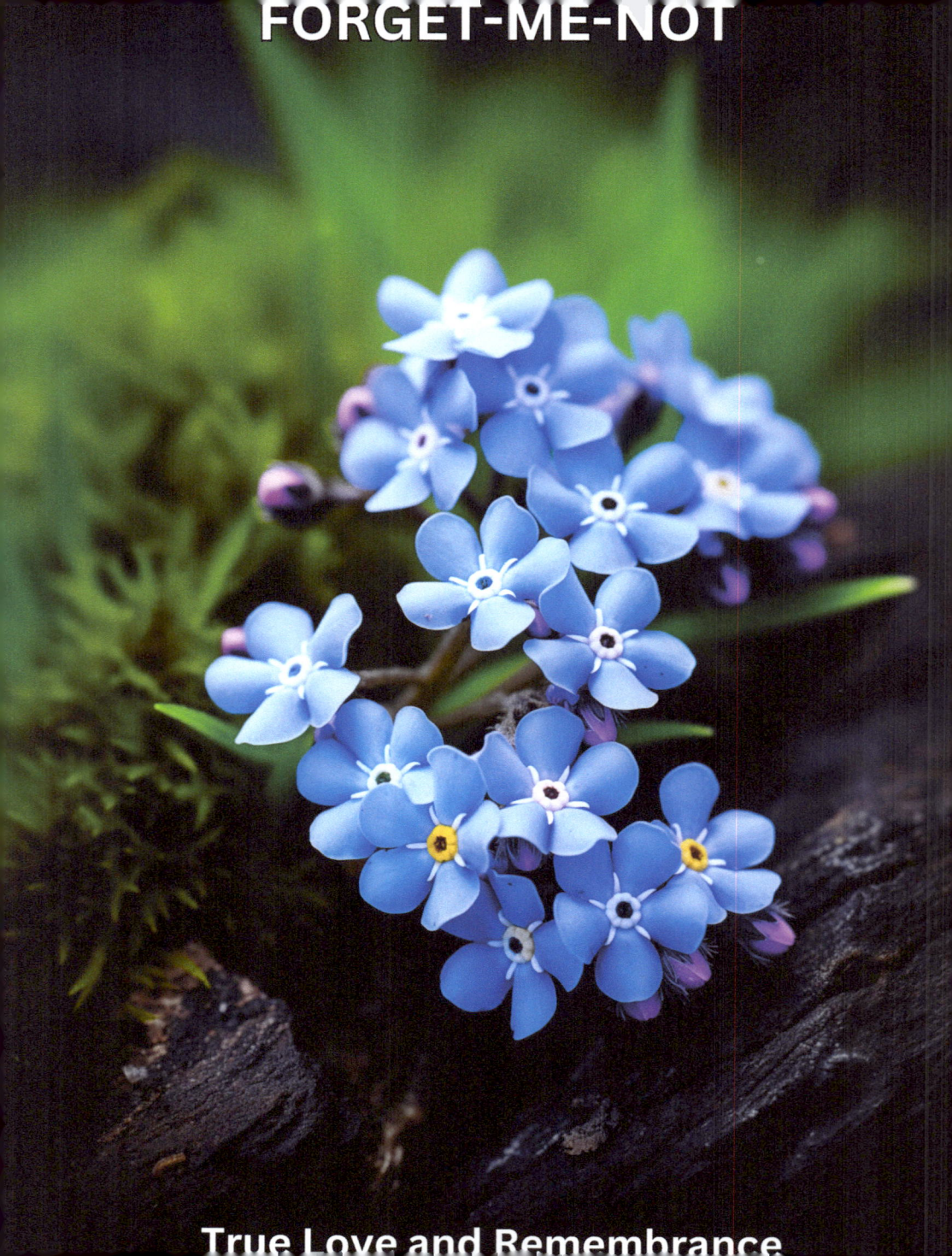

True Love and Remembrance

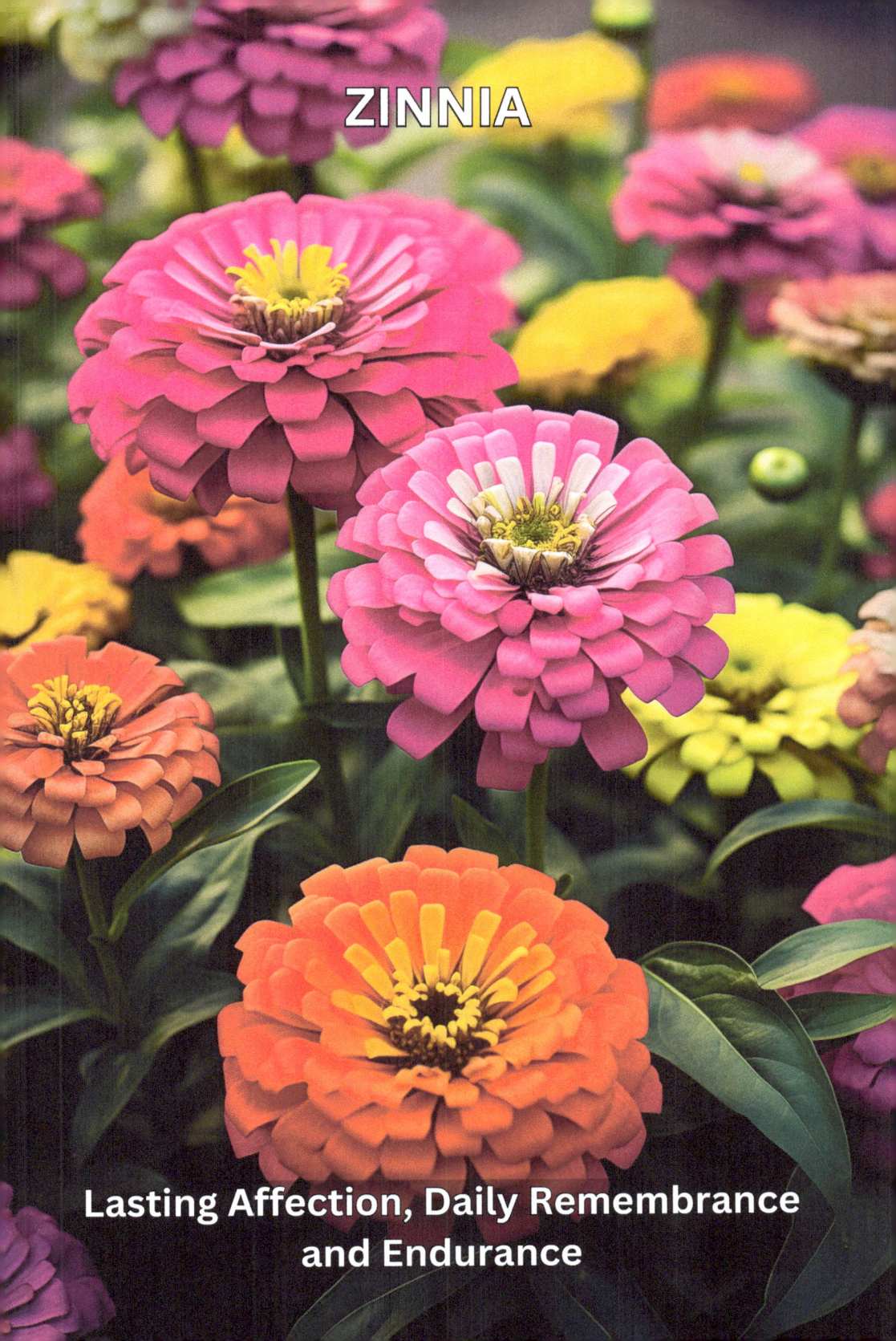

SAGUARO

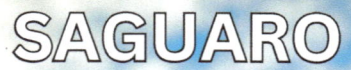

Resilience, Protection and Endurance

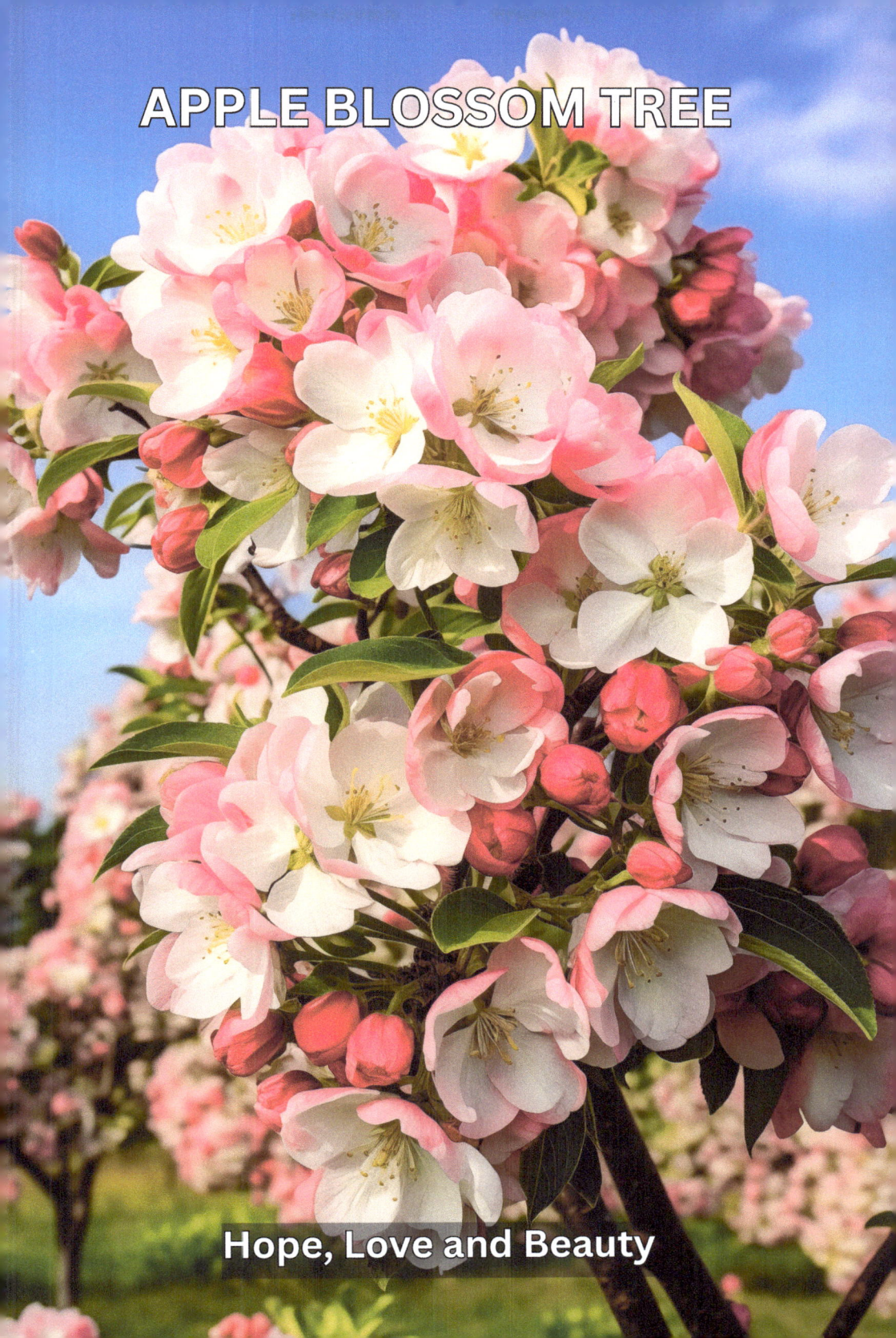

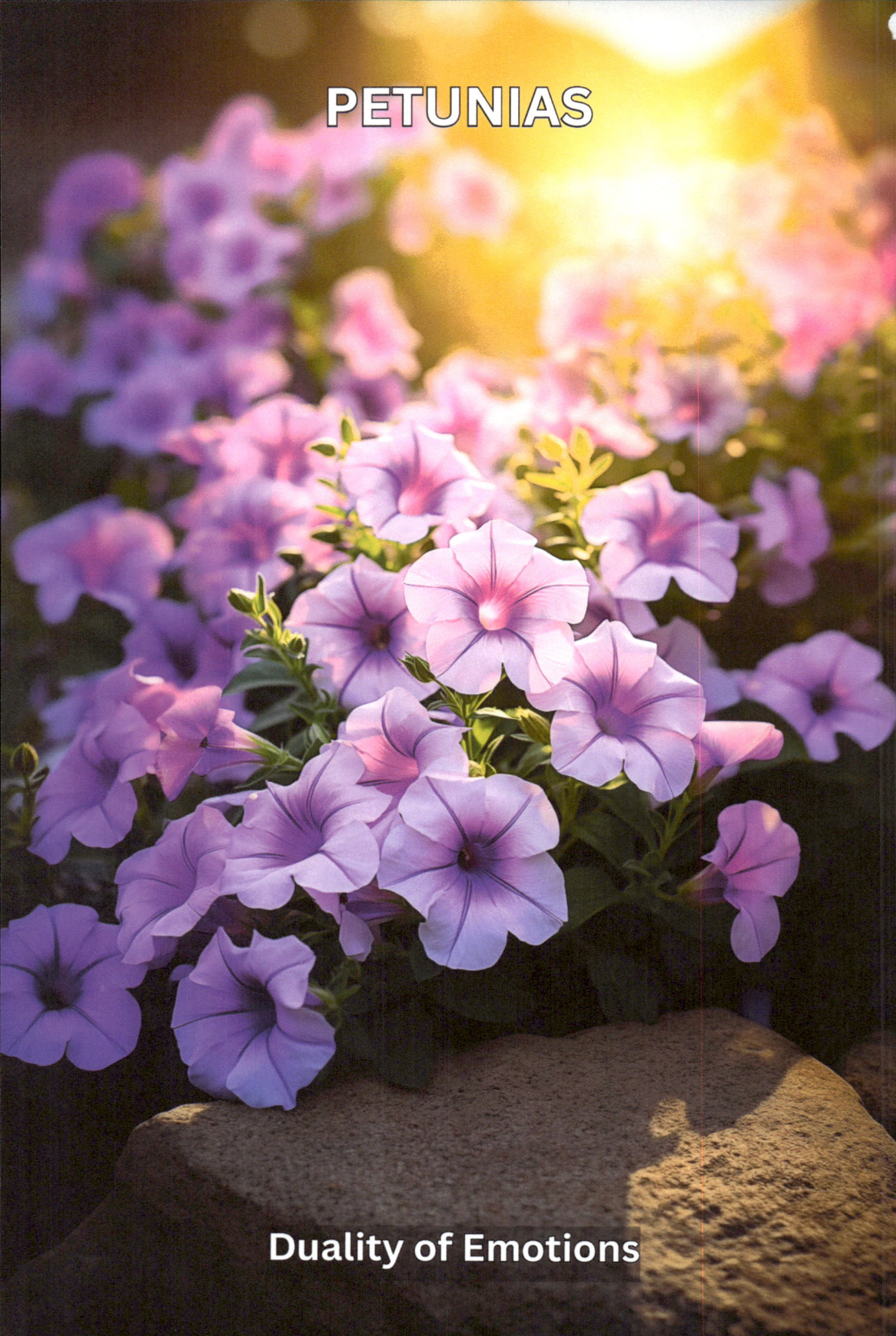

CALIFORNIA POPPY

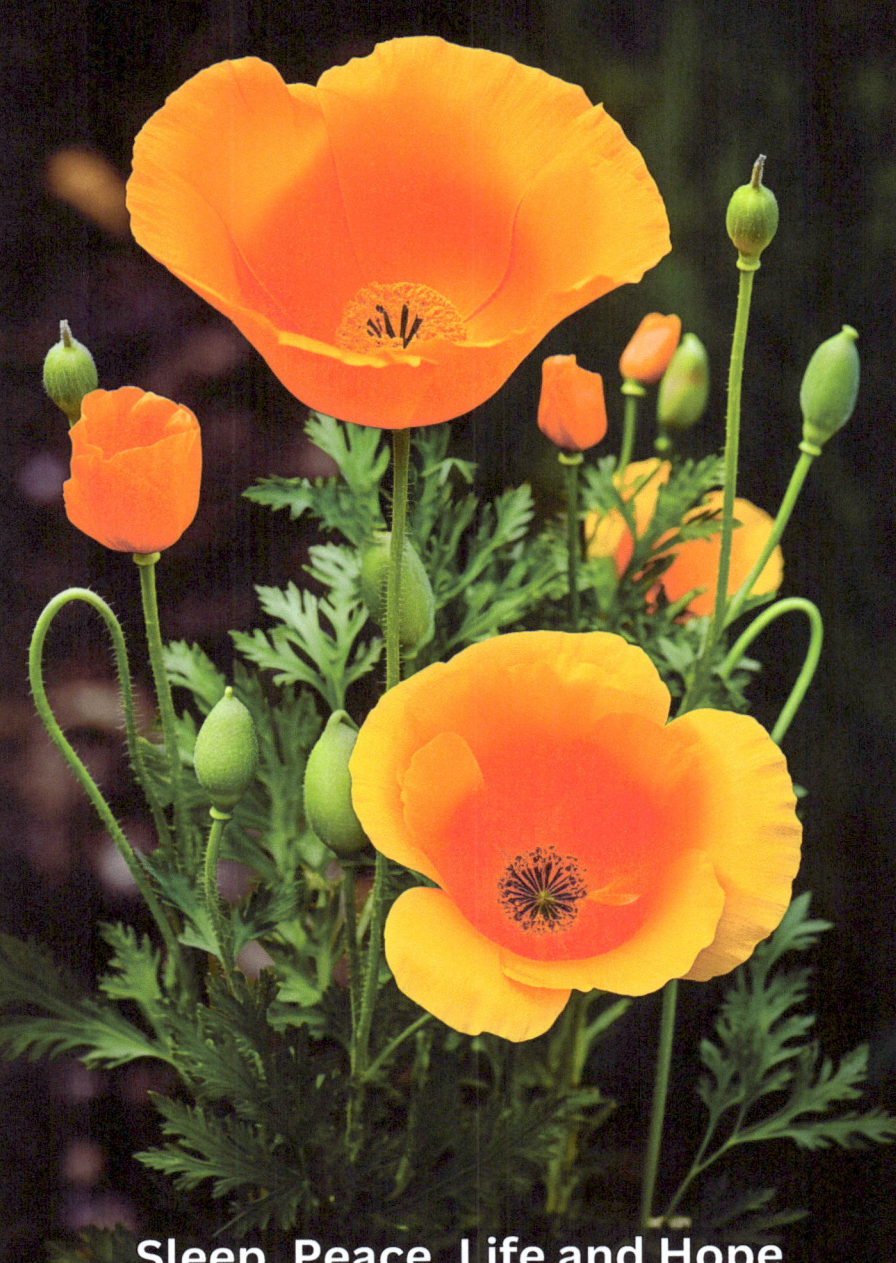

Sleep, Peace, Life and Hope
The State Flower of California

MOUNTAIN LAUREL

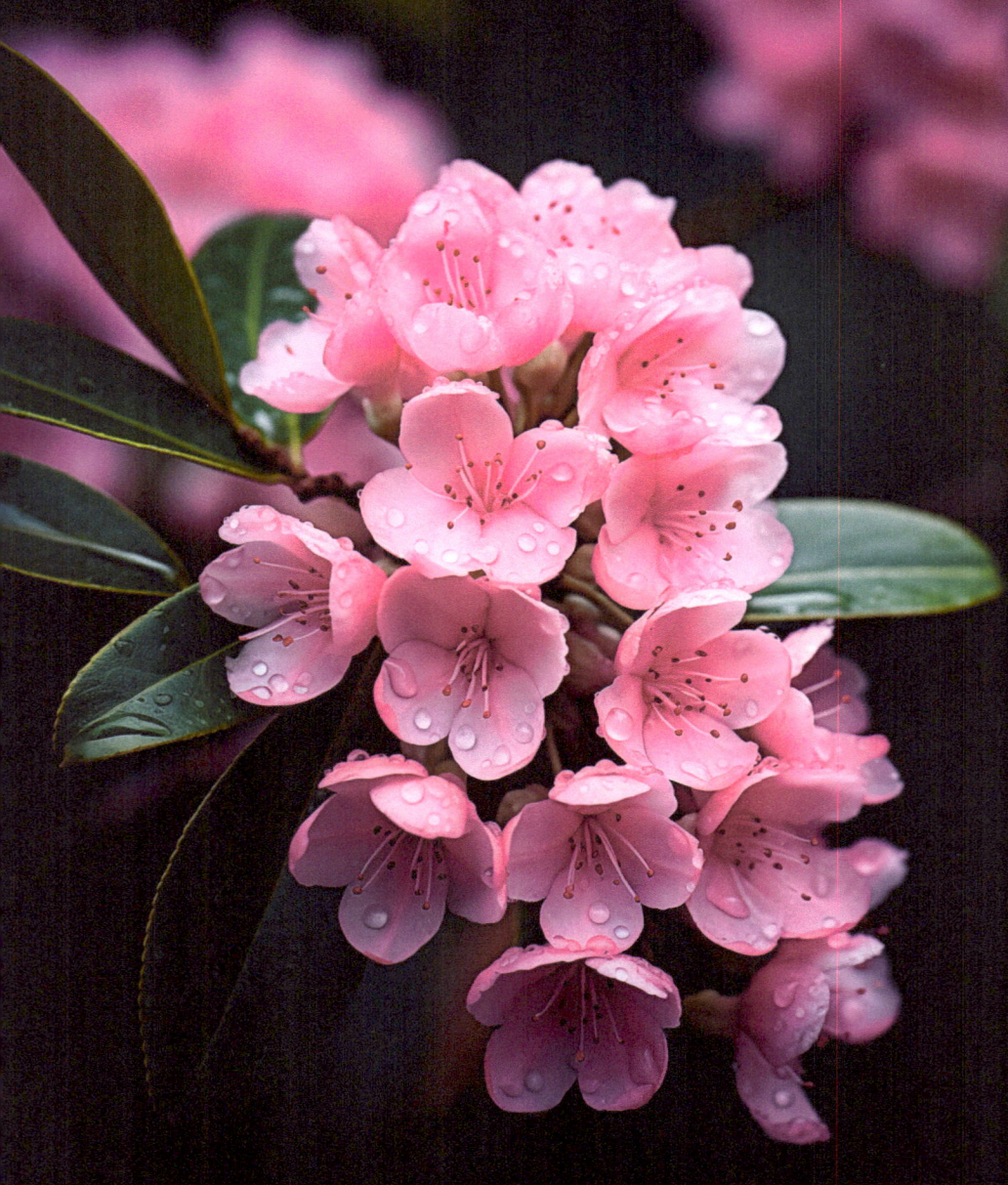

Ambition and Perseverance

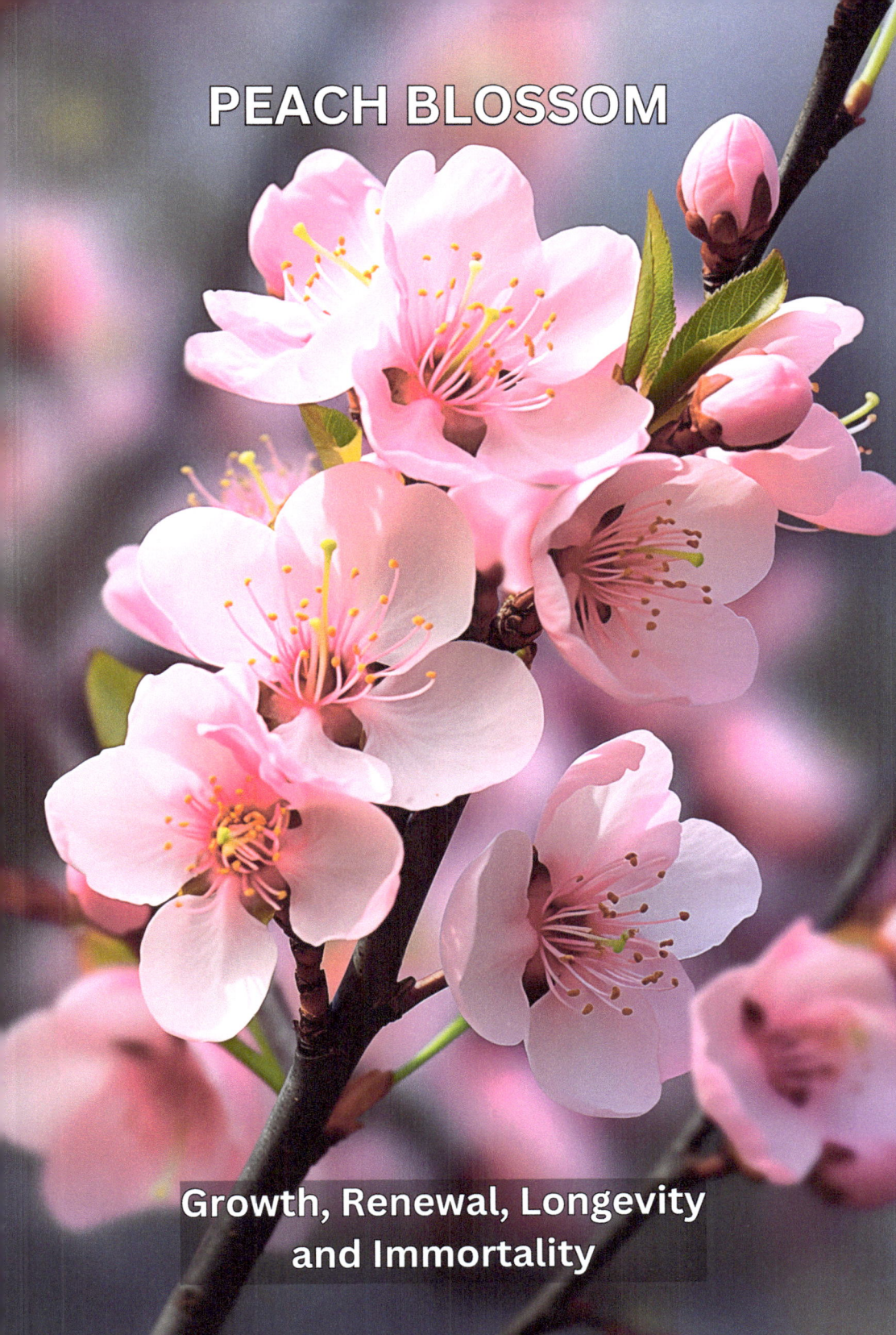

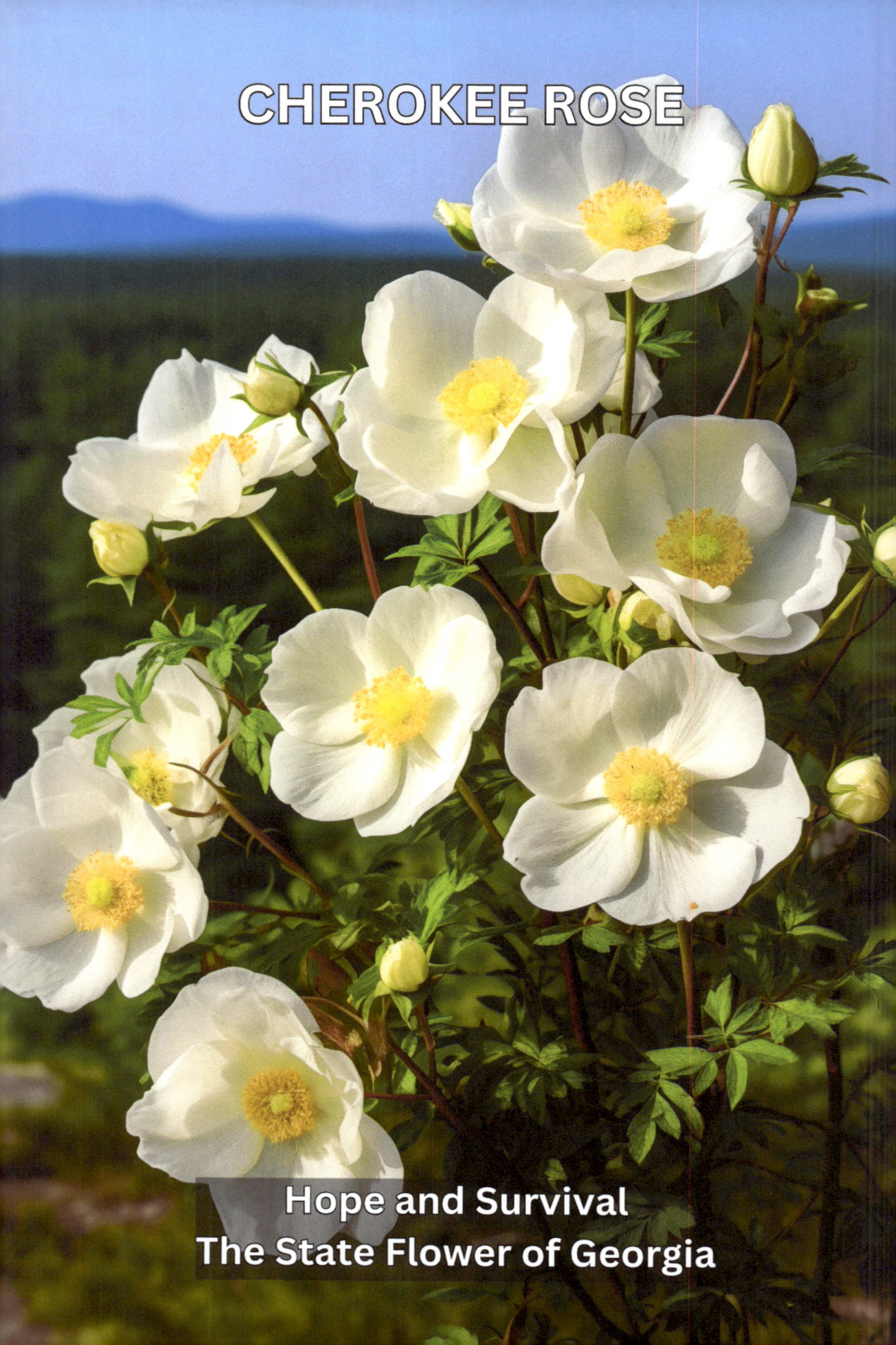

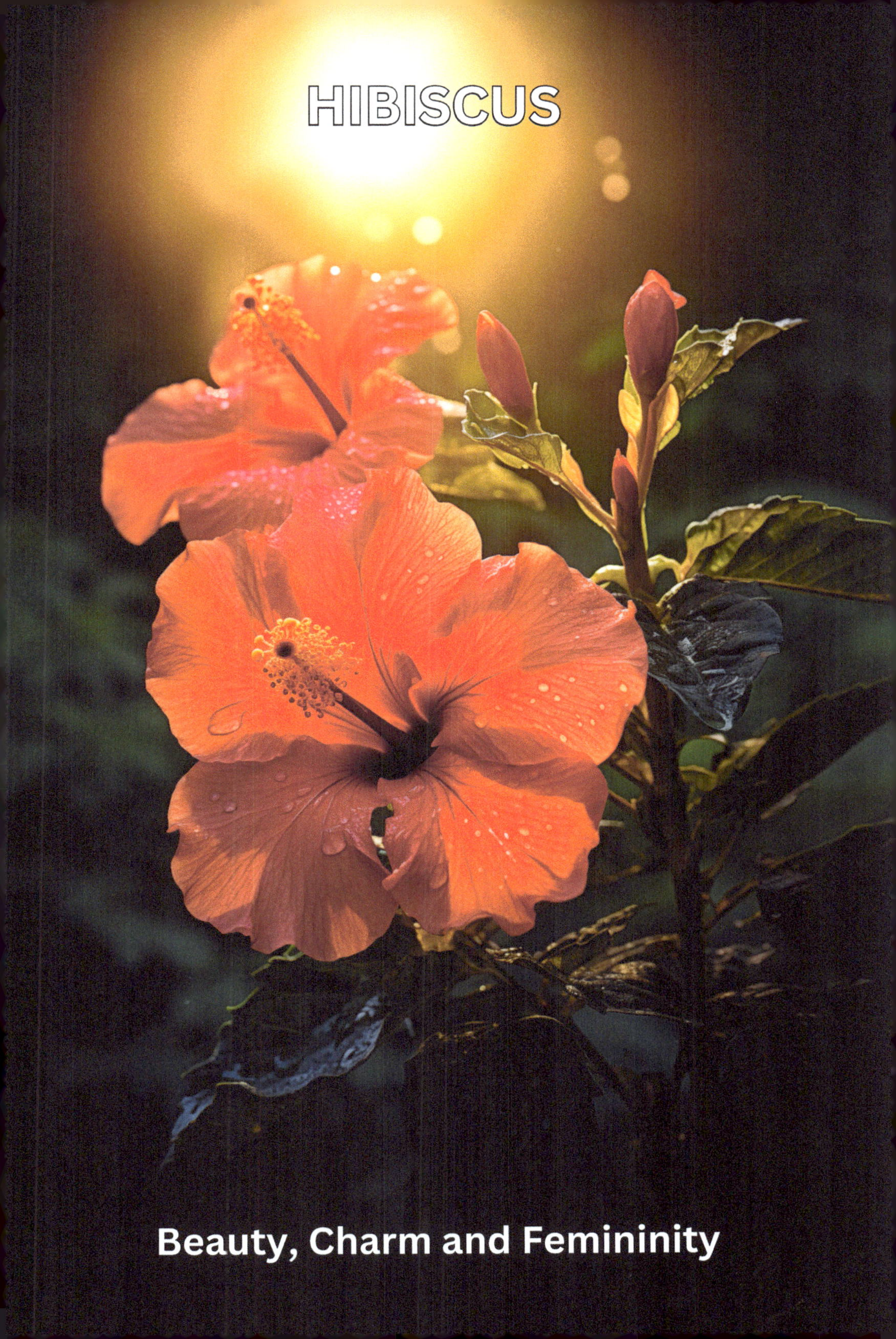

HIBISCUS

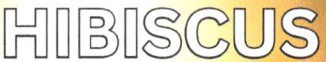

Beauty, Charm and Femininity

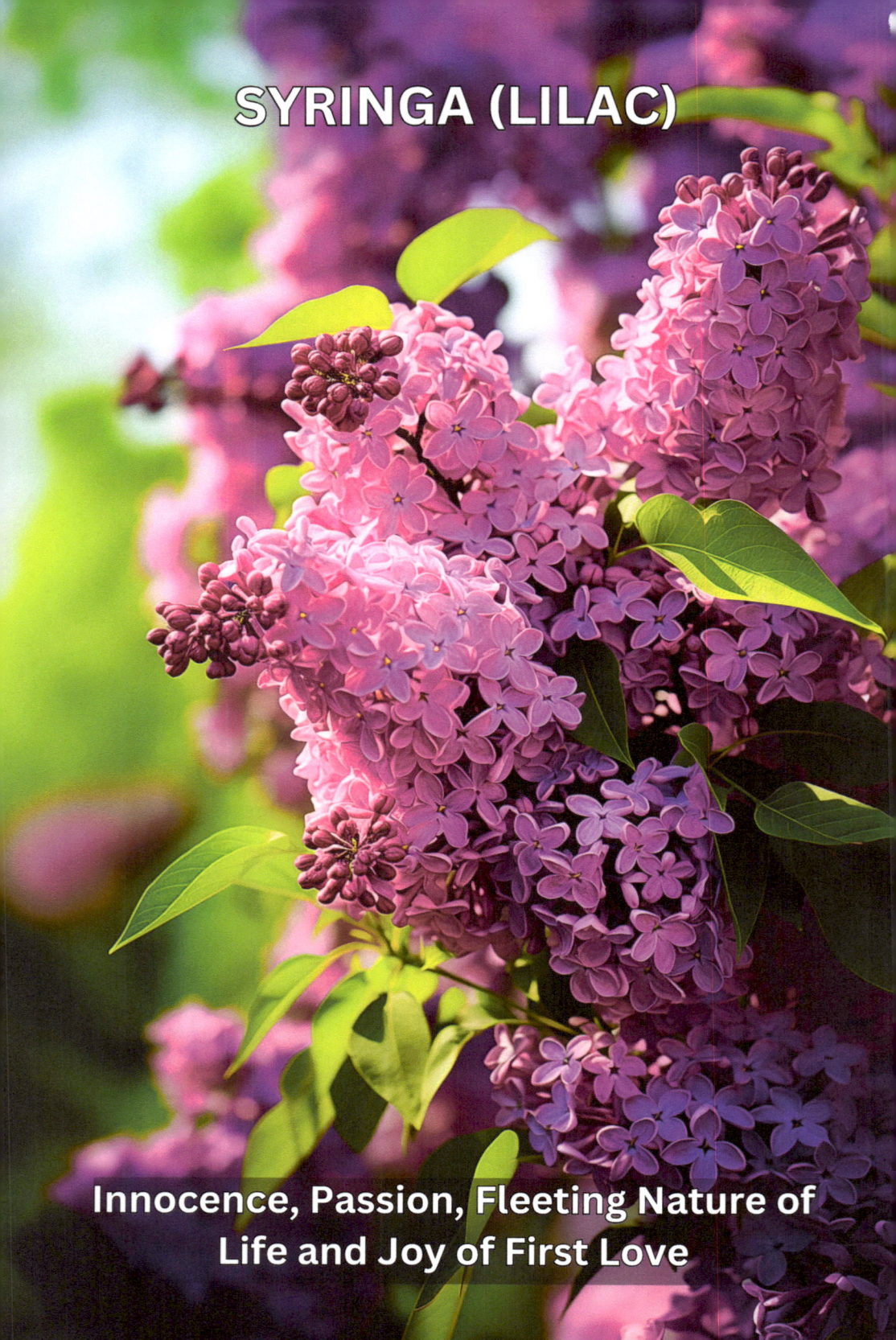

HEPATICA (LIVERLEAF)

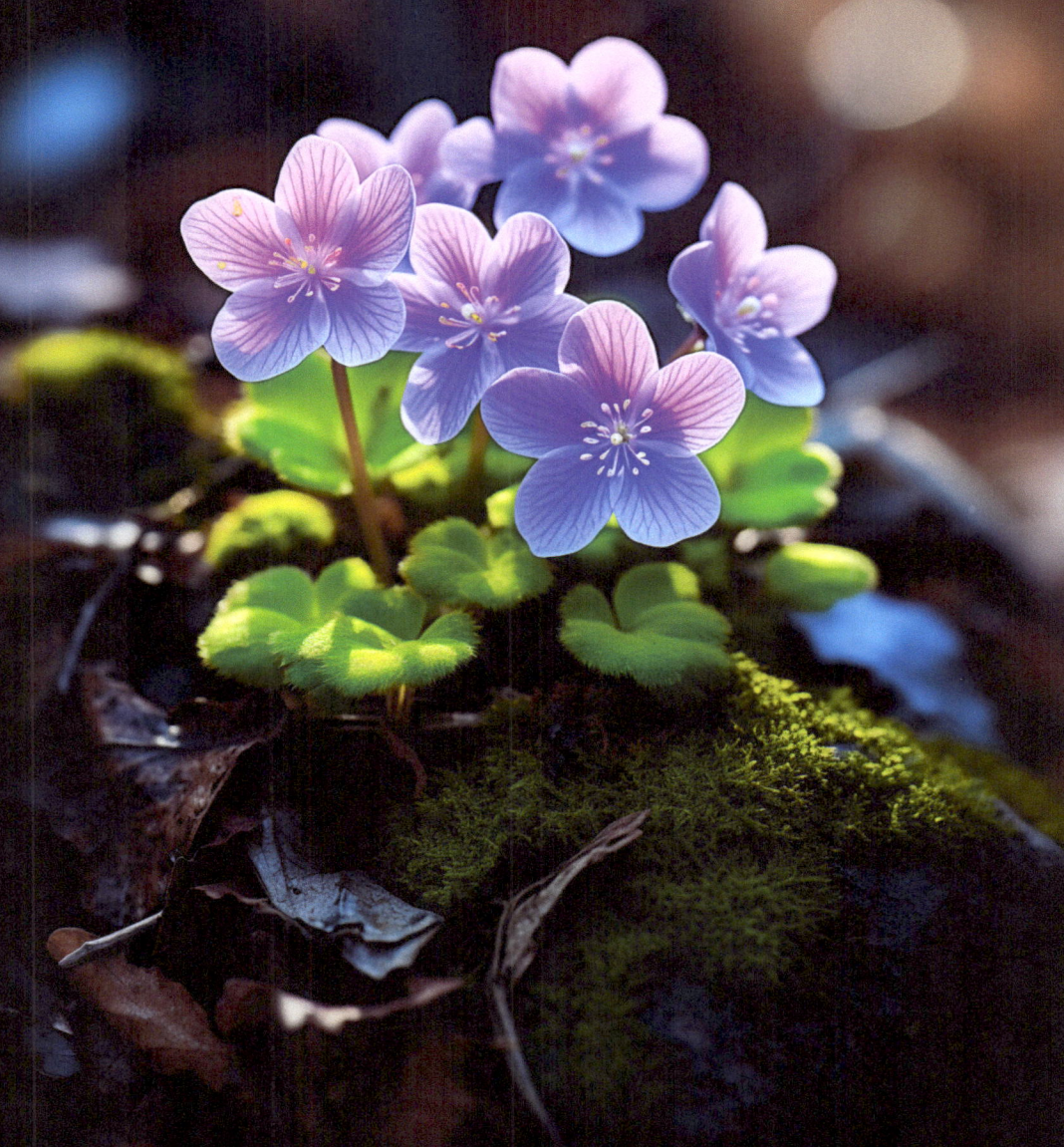

Rebirth, Confidence and Protection

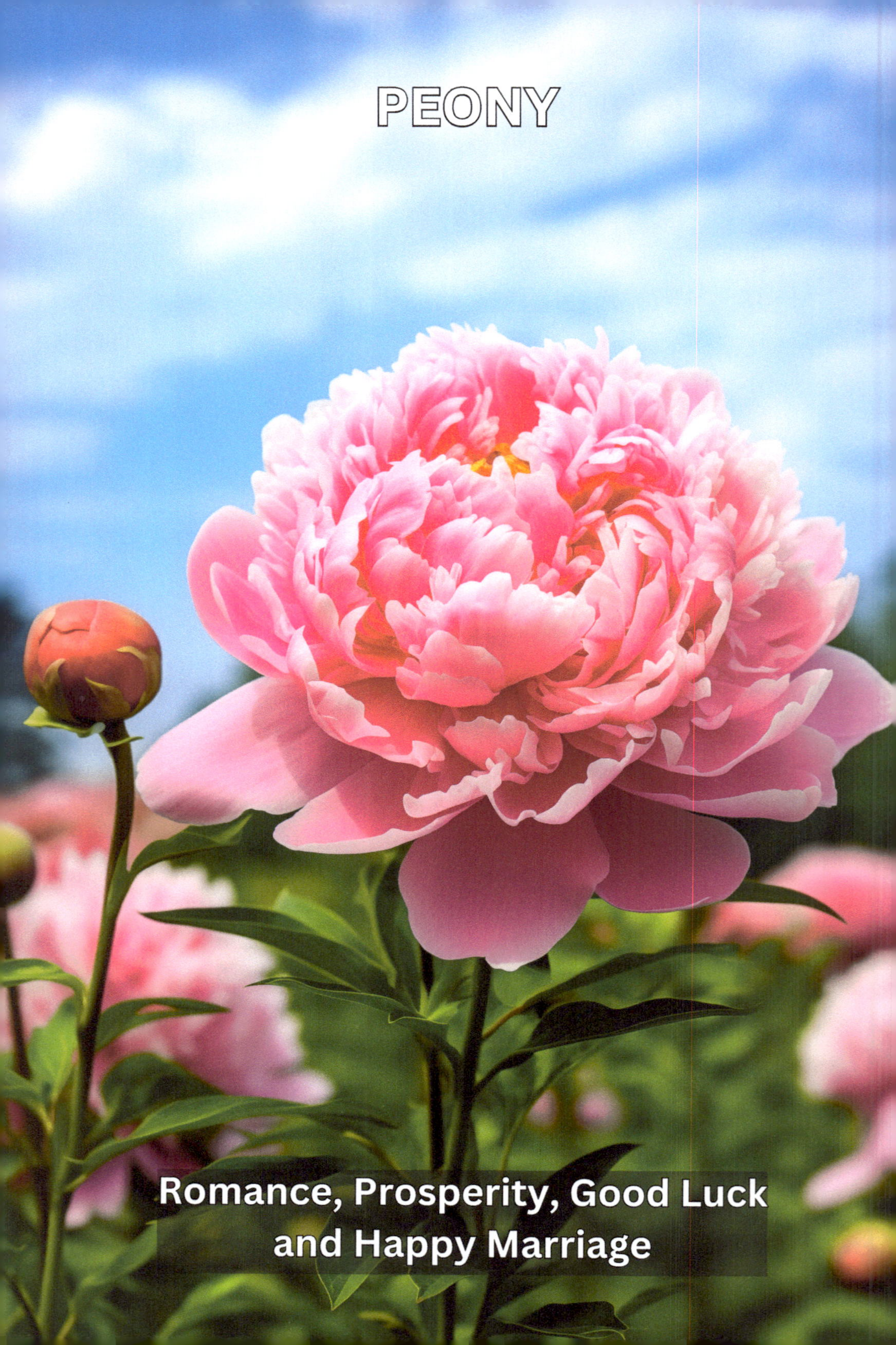

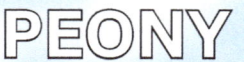

PEONY

Romance, Prosperity, Good Luck and Happy Marriage

WILD ROSE

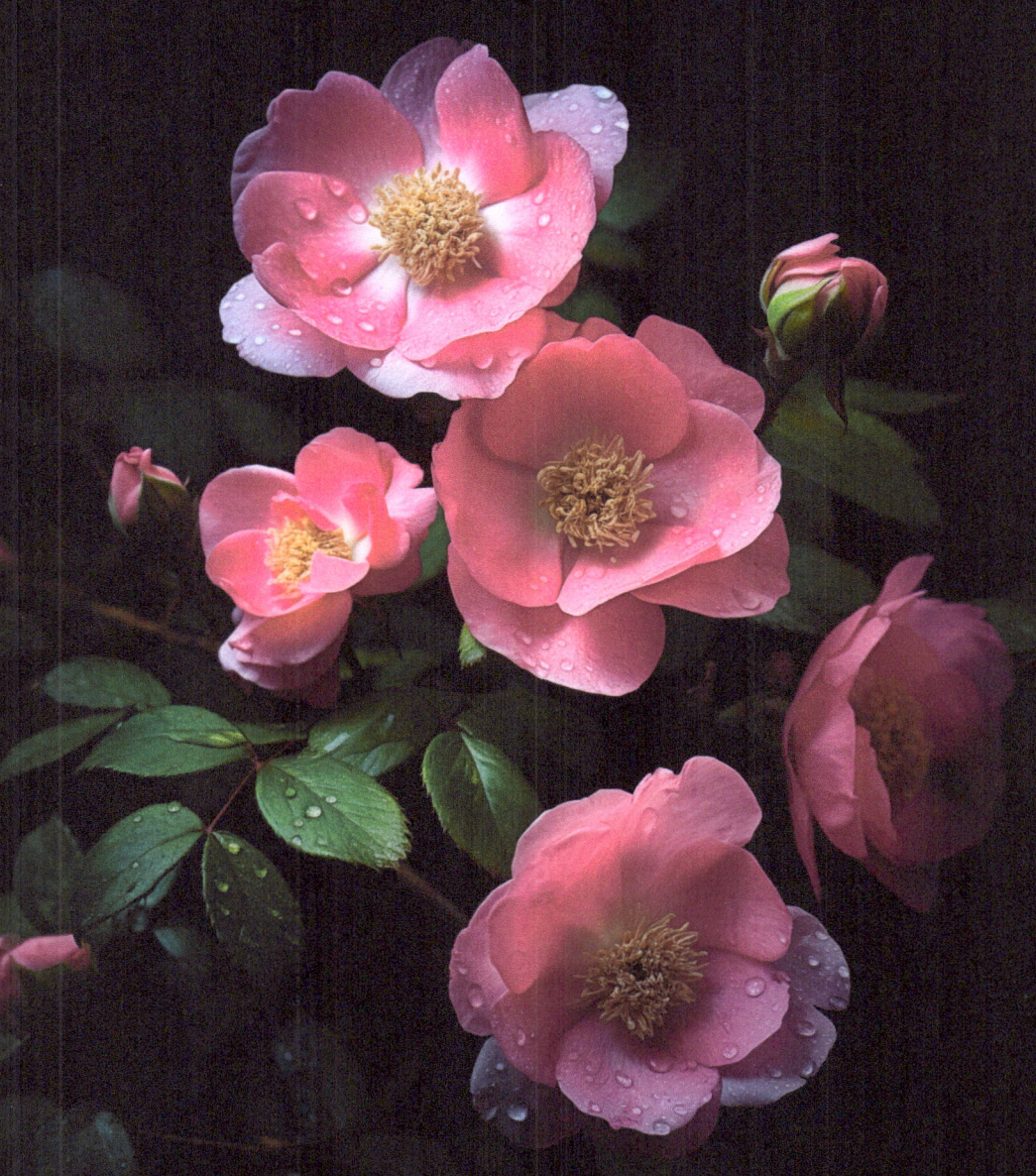

Simplicity, Endurance and Spontaneous Beauty

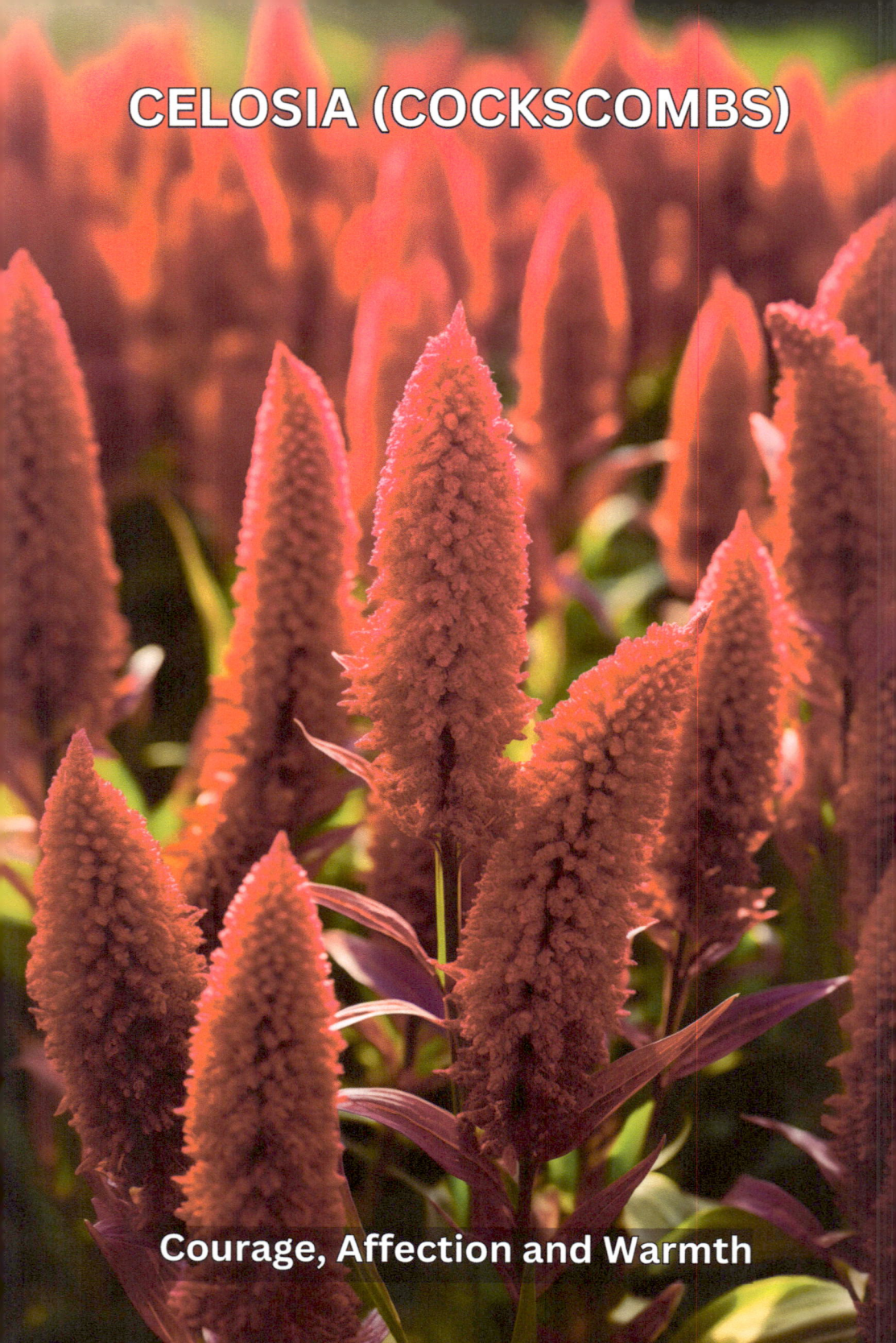

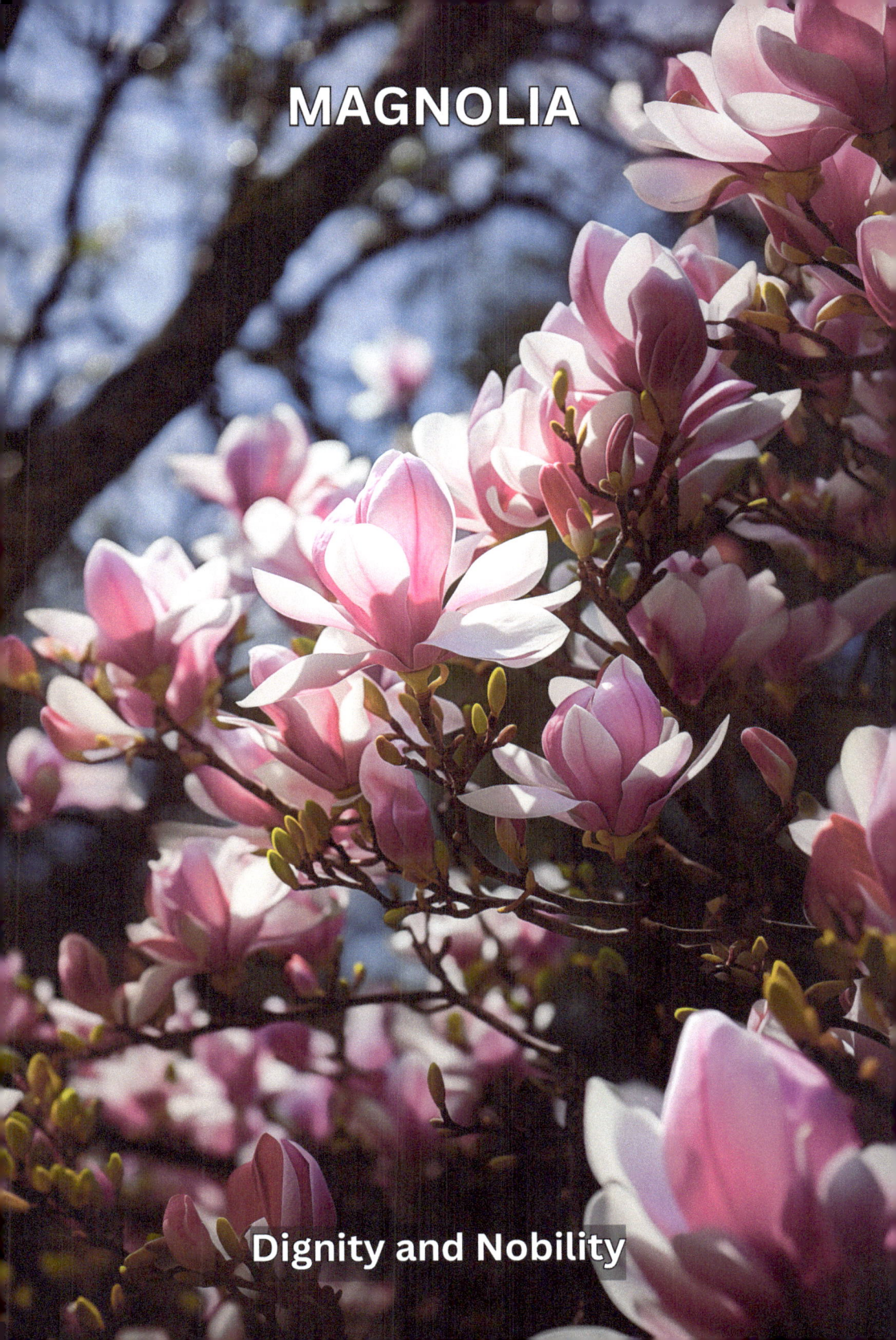

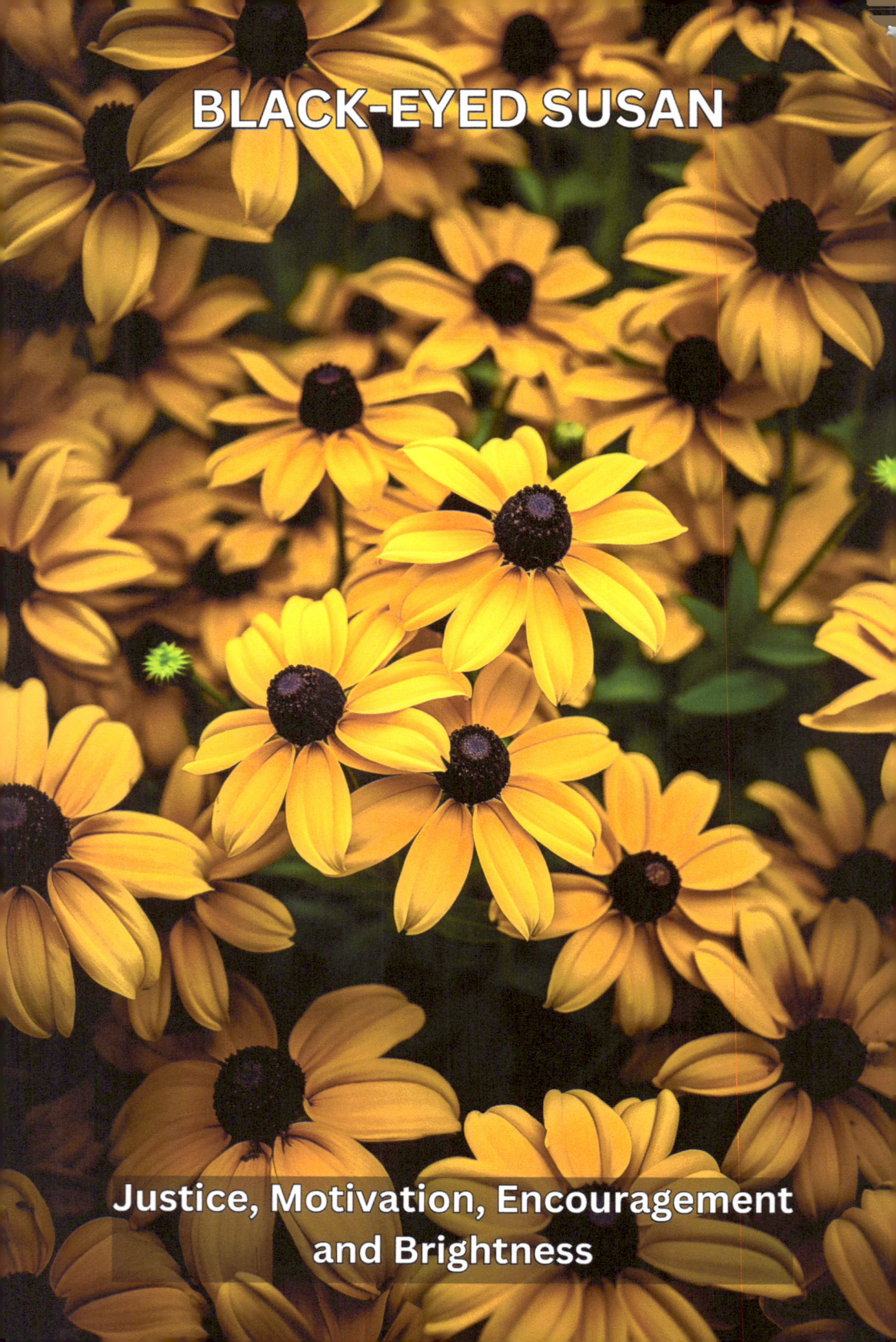

LARGE BITTERCRESS

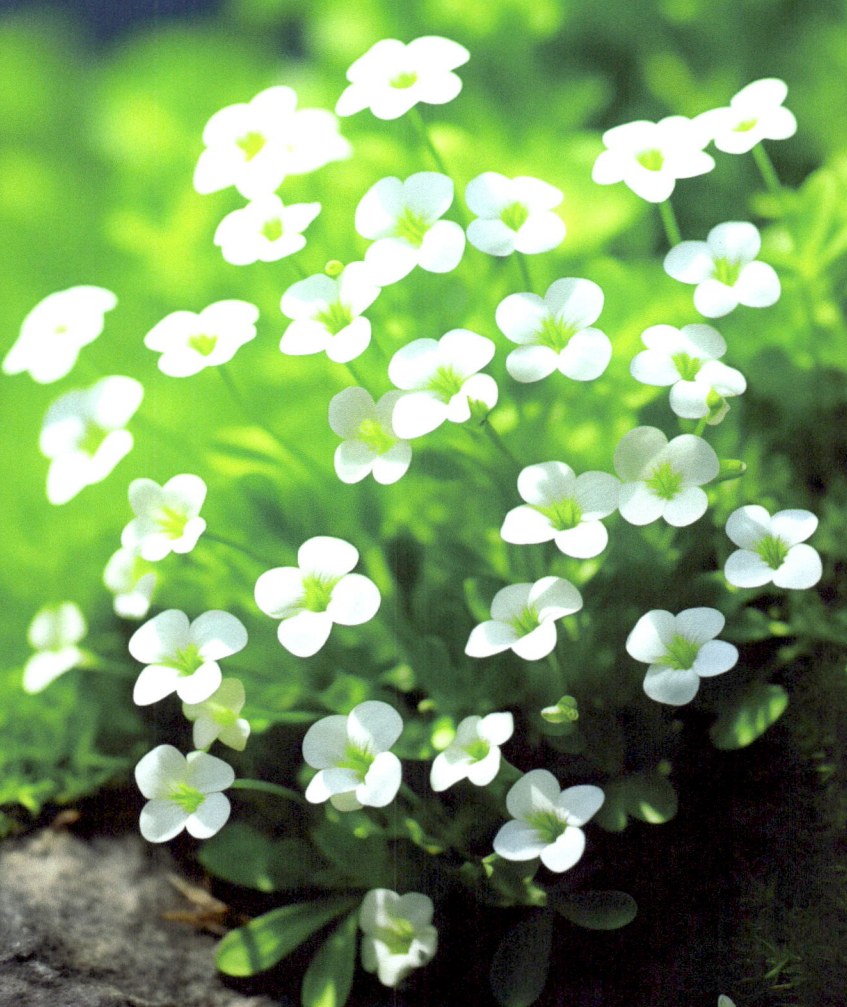

Hardiness and Adaptability

GERANIUMS

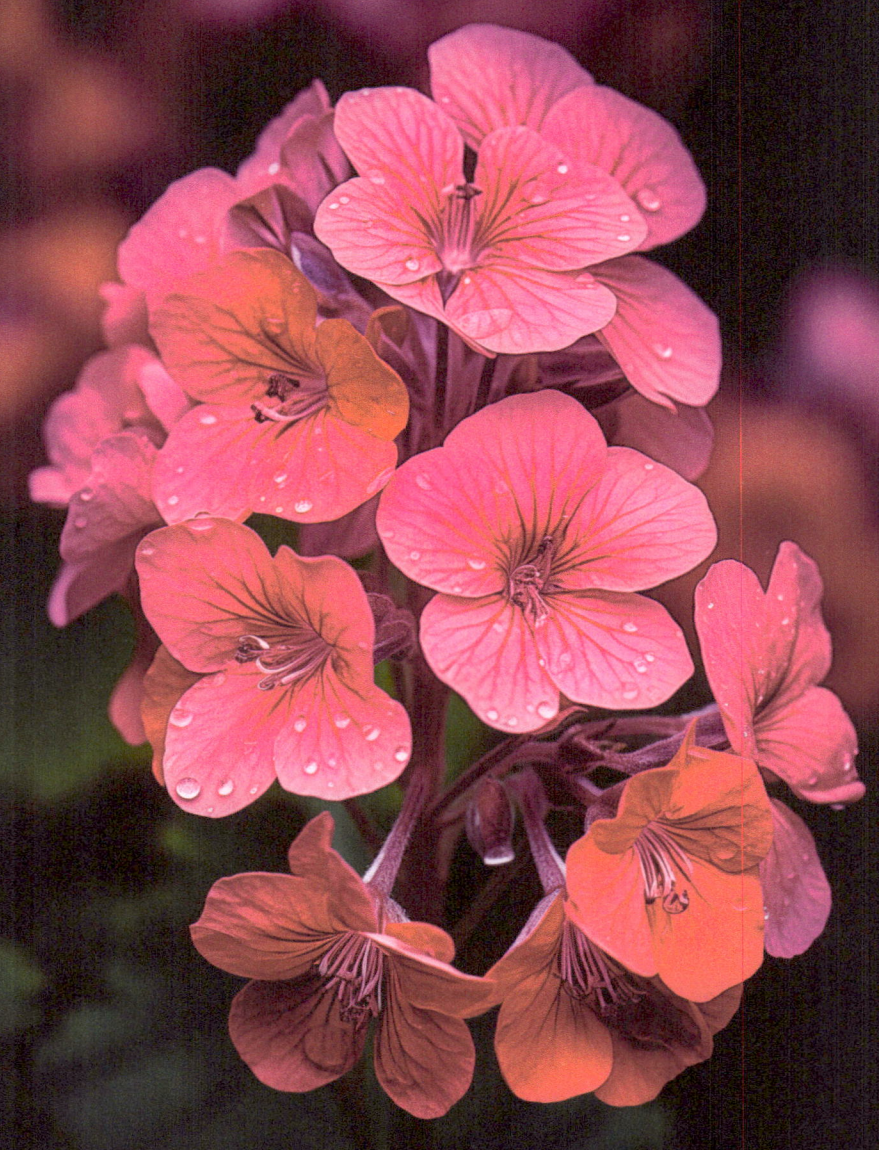

Friendship and Positive Emotions

WHITE HAWTHORN BLOSSOM

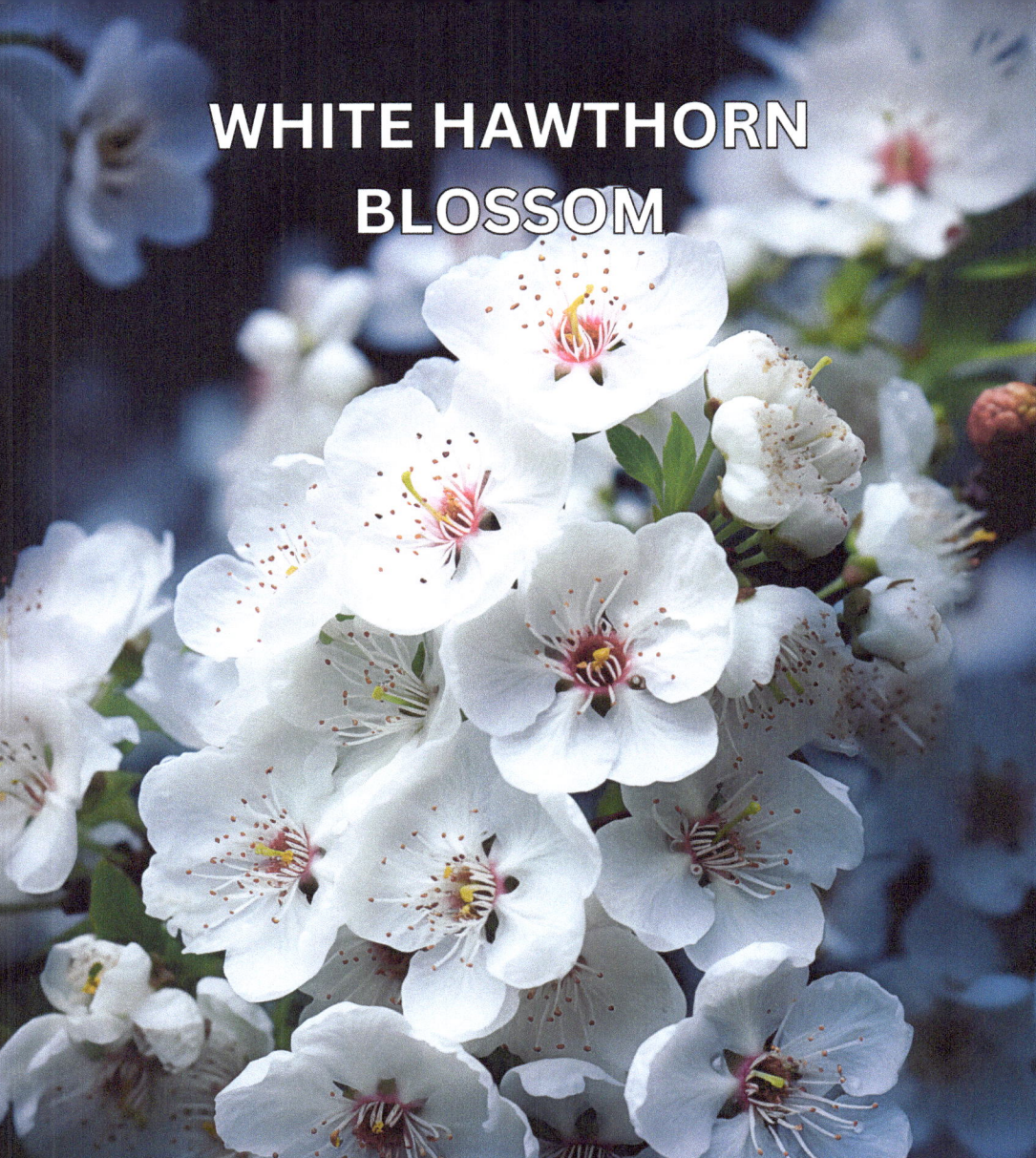

Happiness, Good Fortune, Hope and Protection

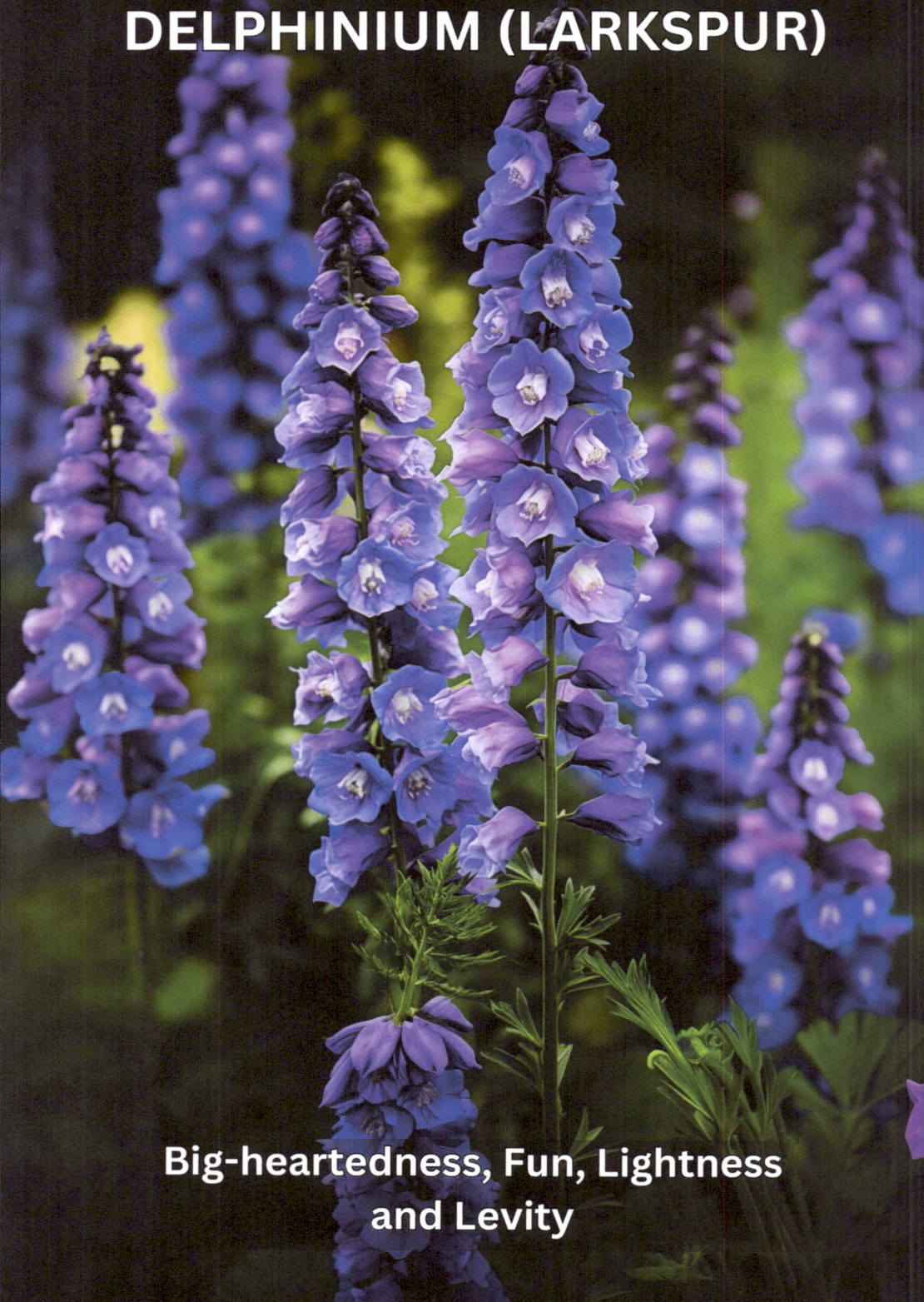
DELPHINIUM (LARKSPUR)

Big-heartedness, Fun, Lightness and Levity

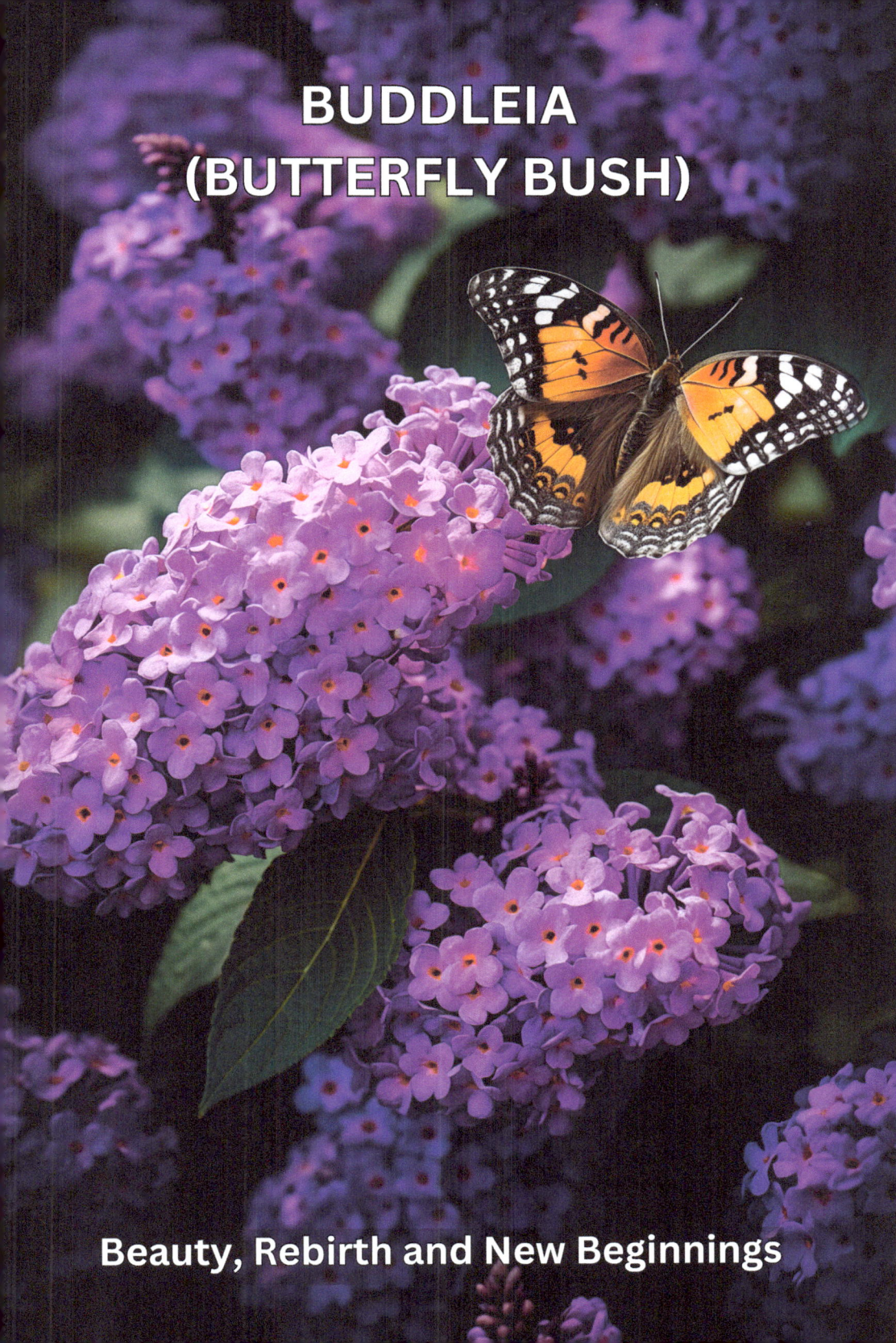

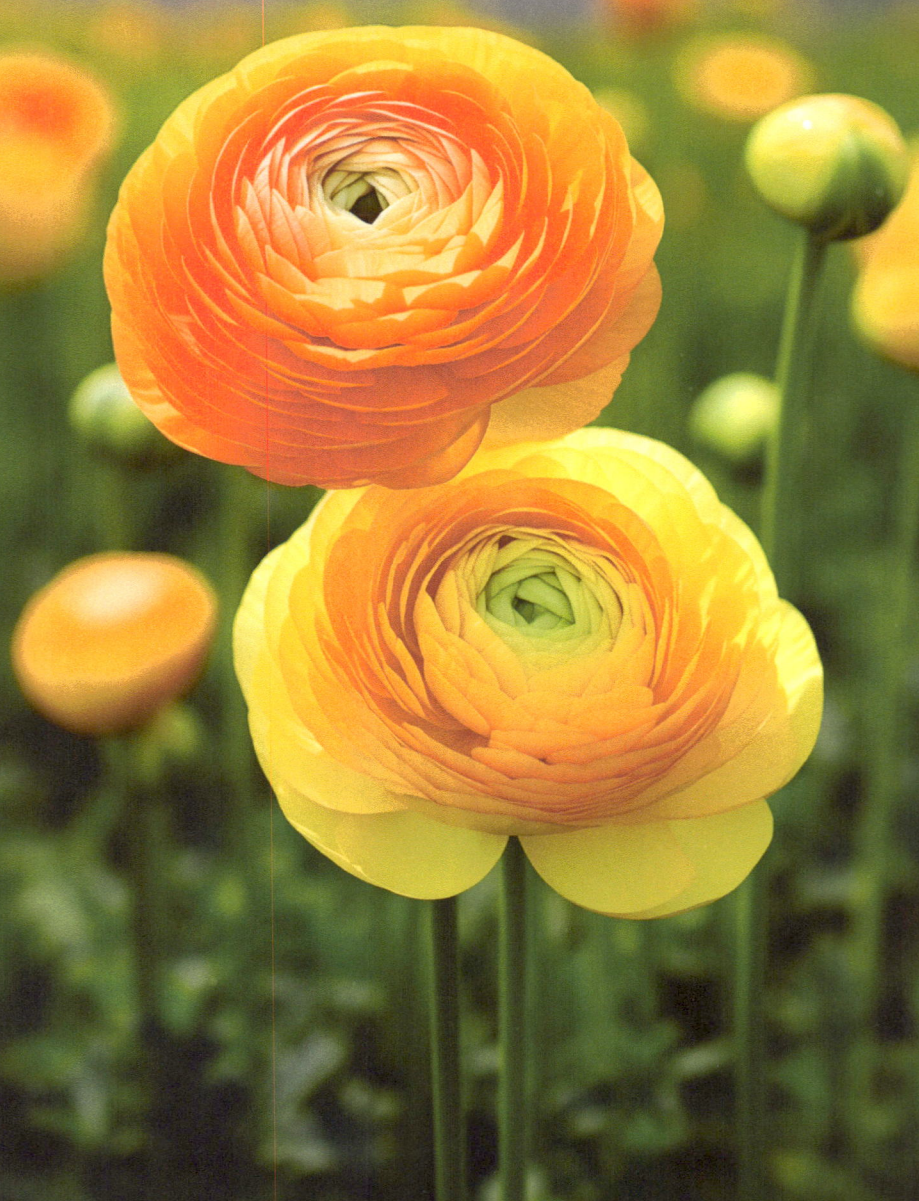

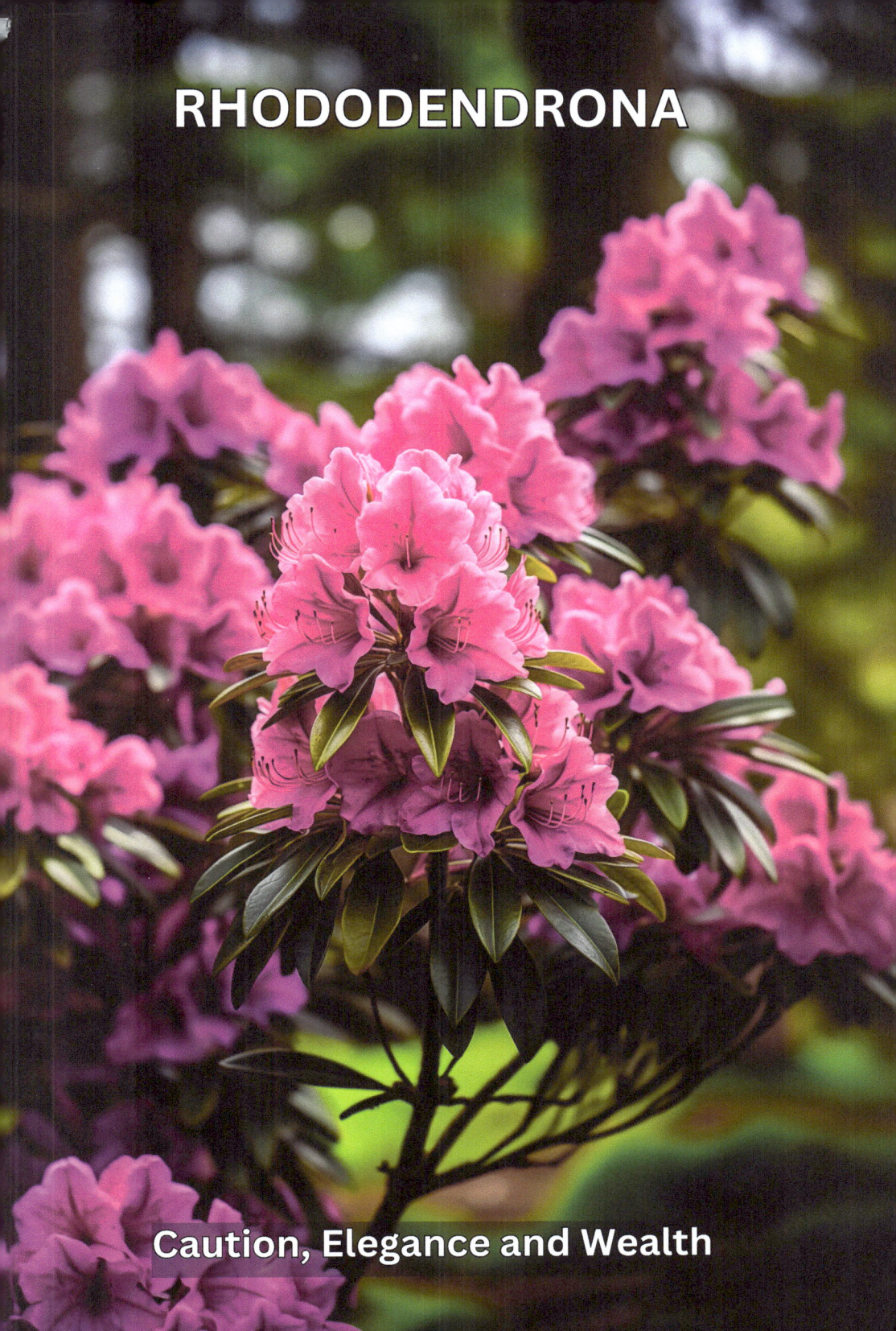

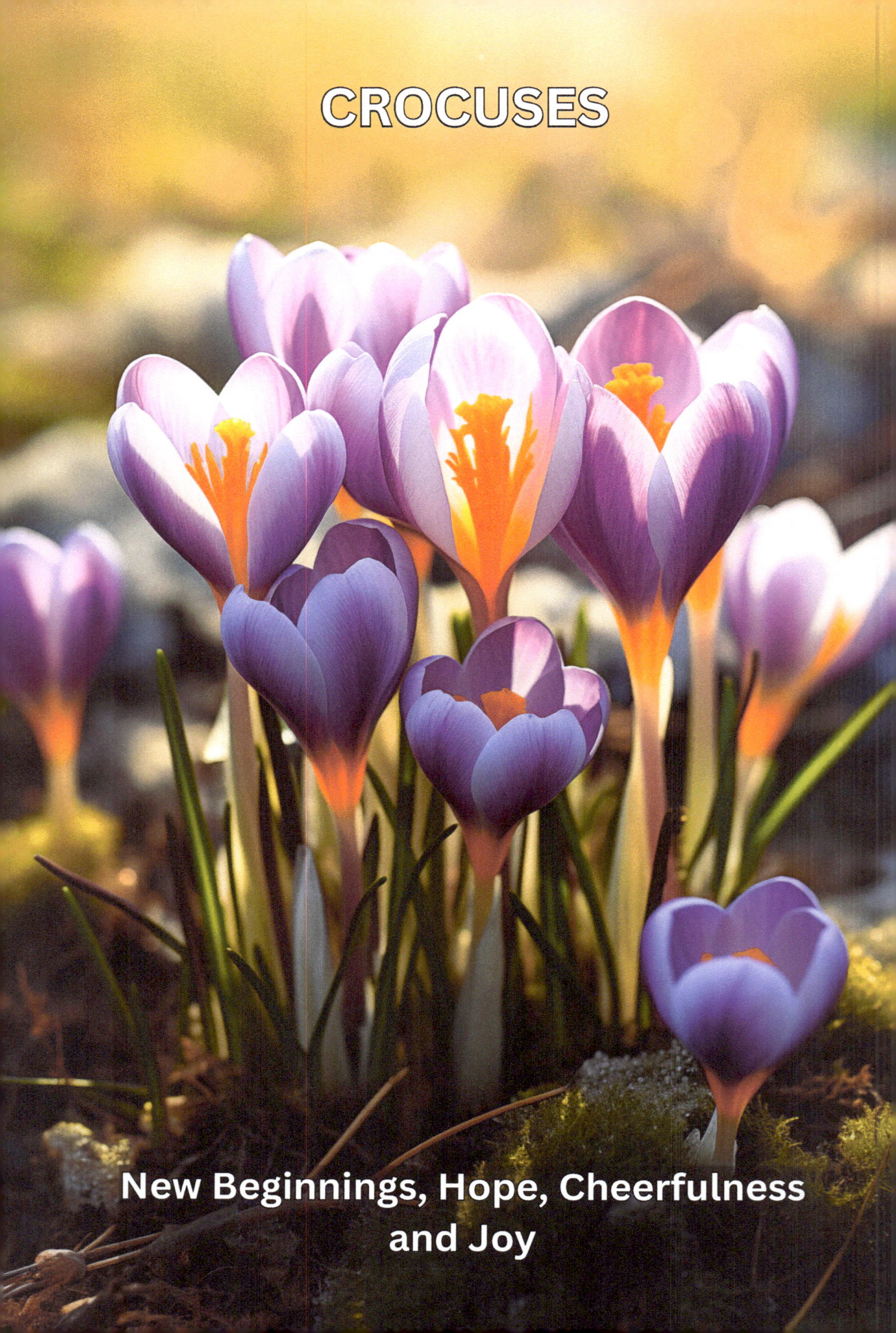

CROCUSES

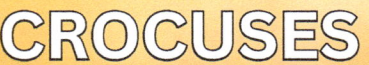

New Beginnings, Hope, Cheerfulness and Joy

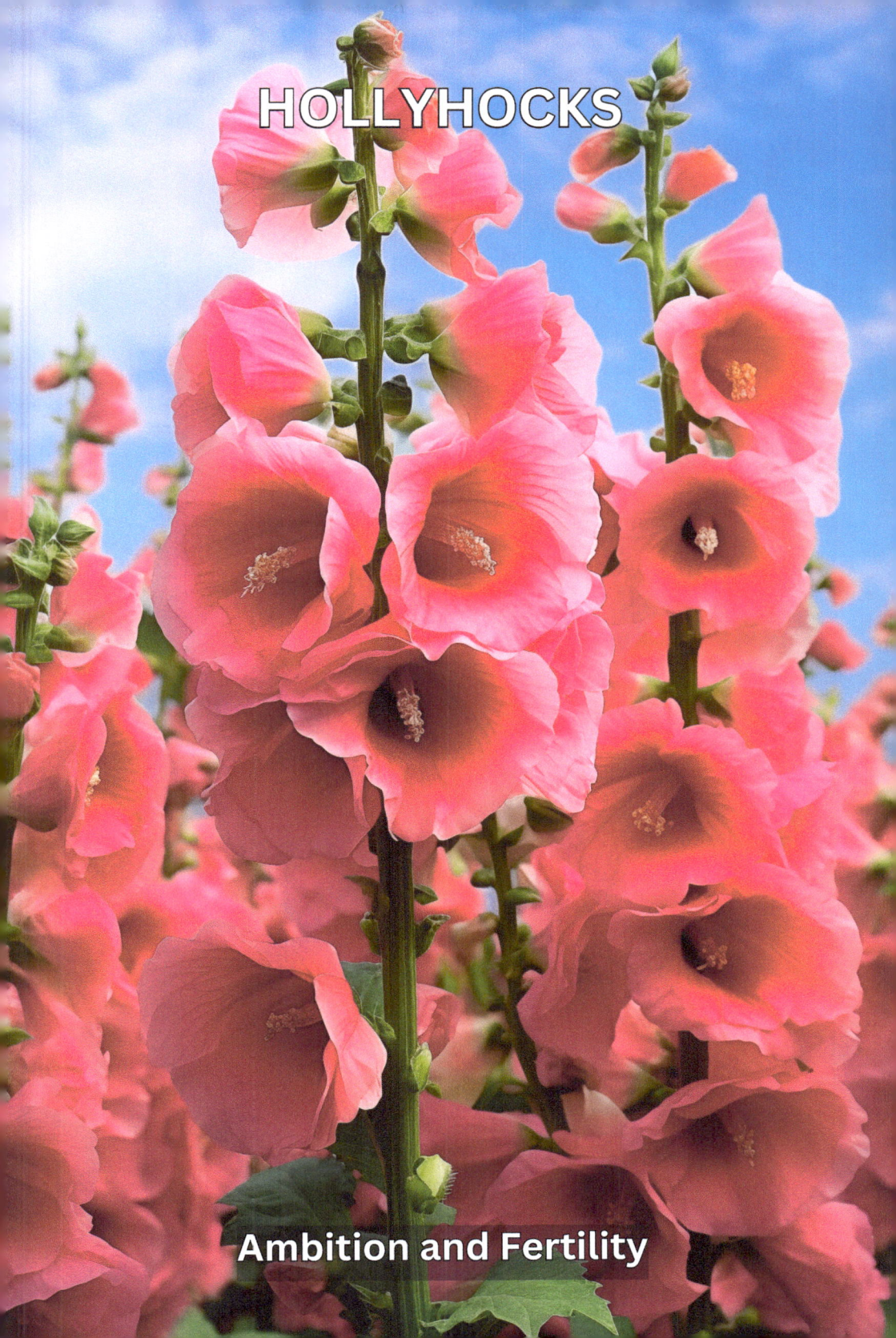

FOXGLOVES

Protection, Magic and Folklore

FREESIAS

Friendship, Thoughtfulness, Trust and Innocence

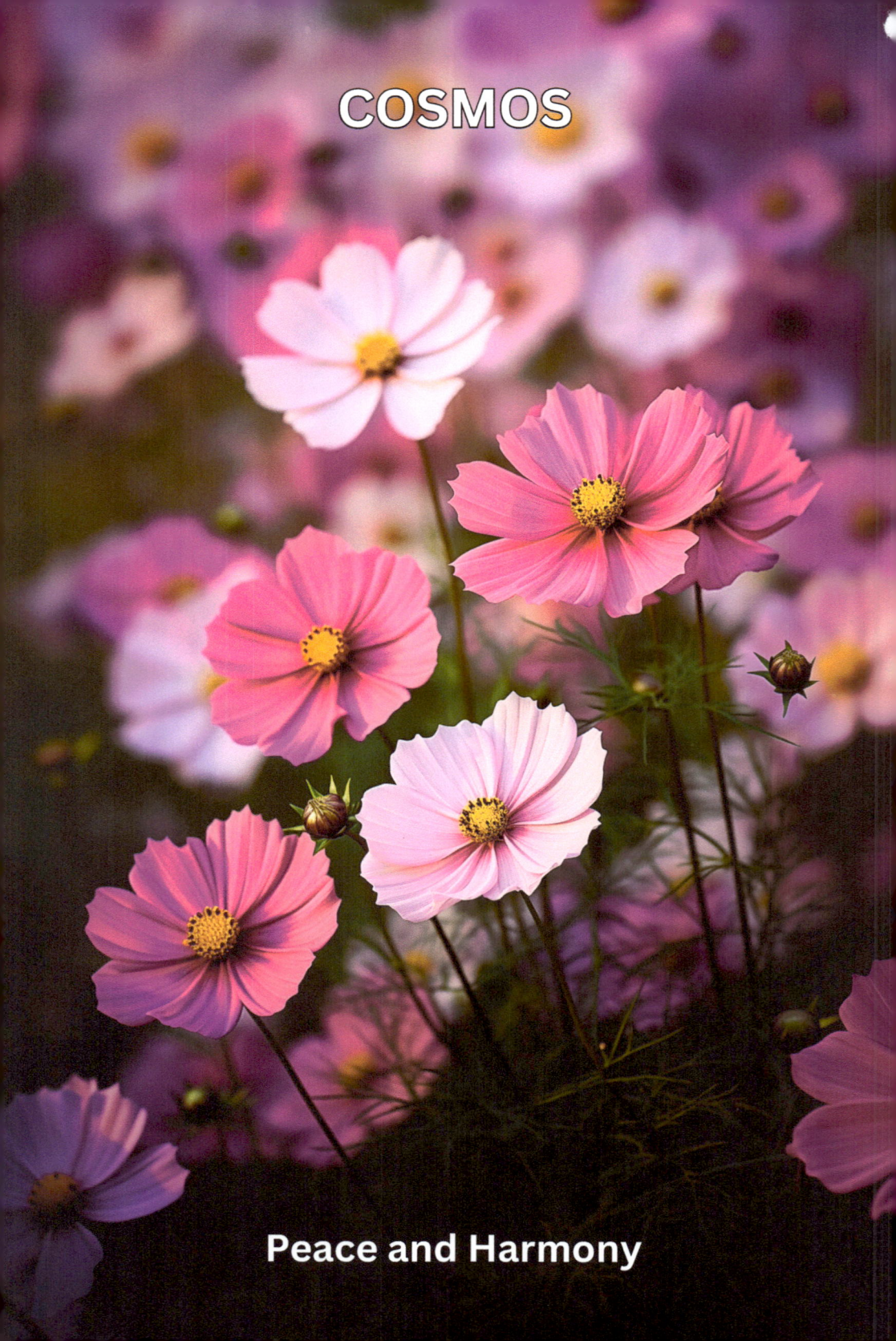

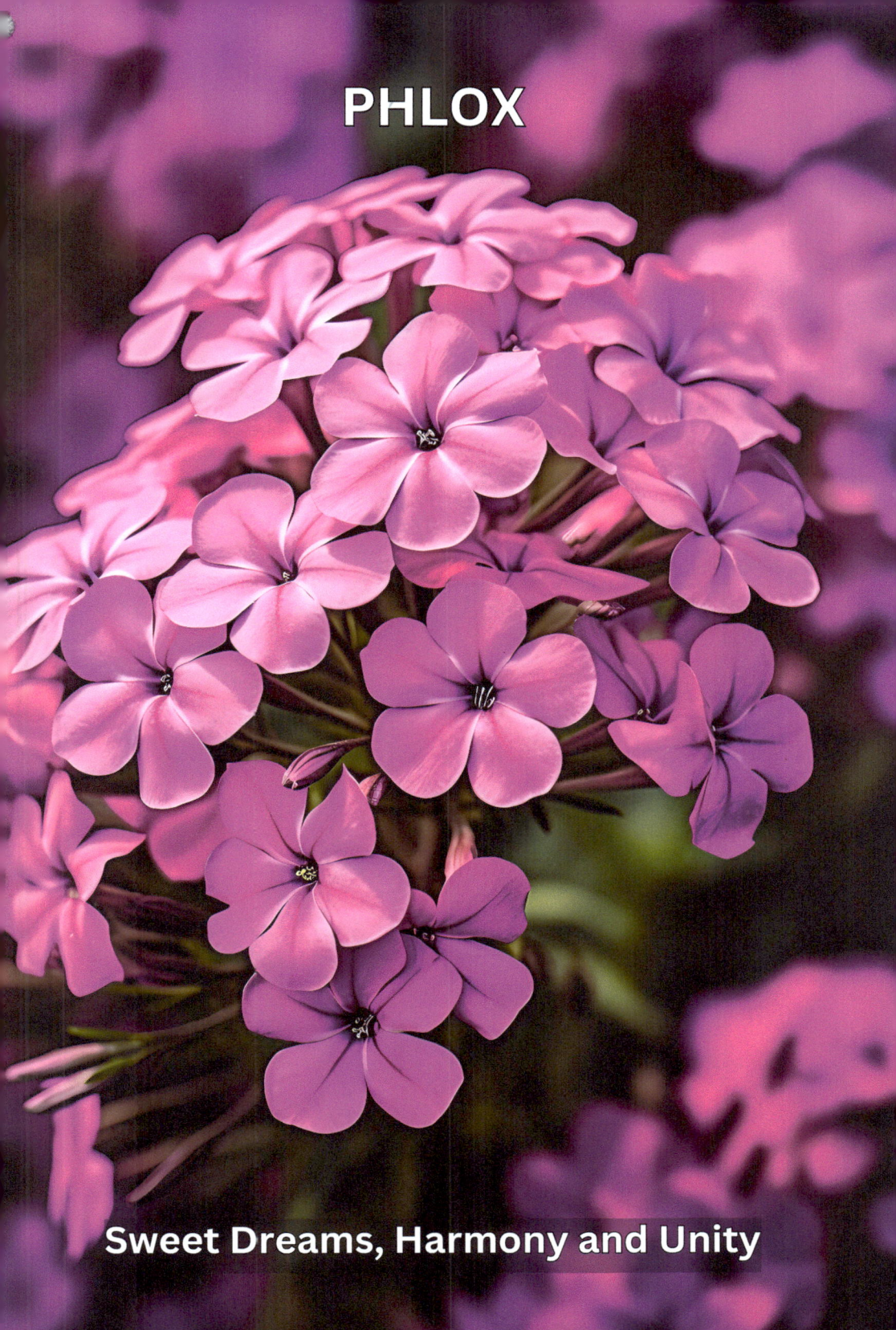

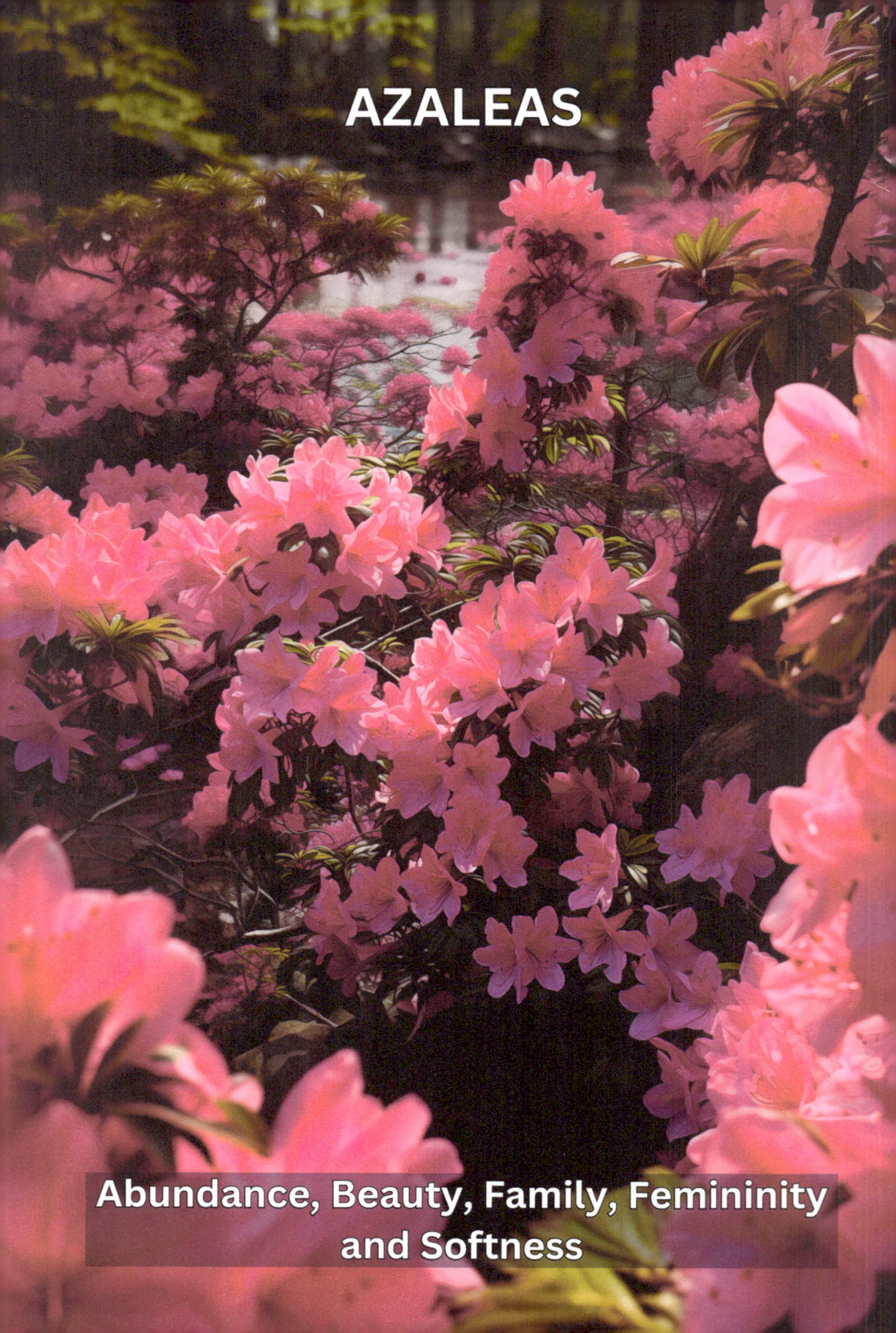

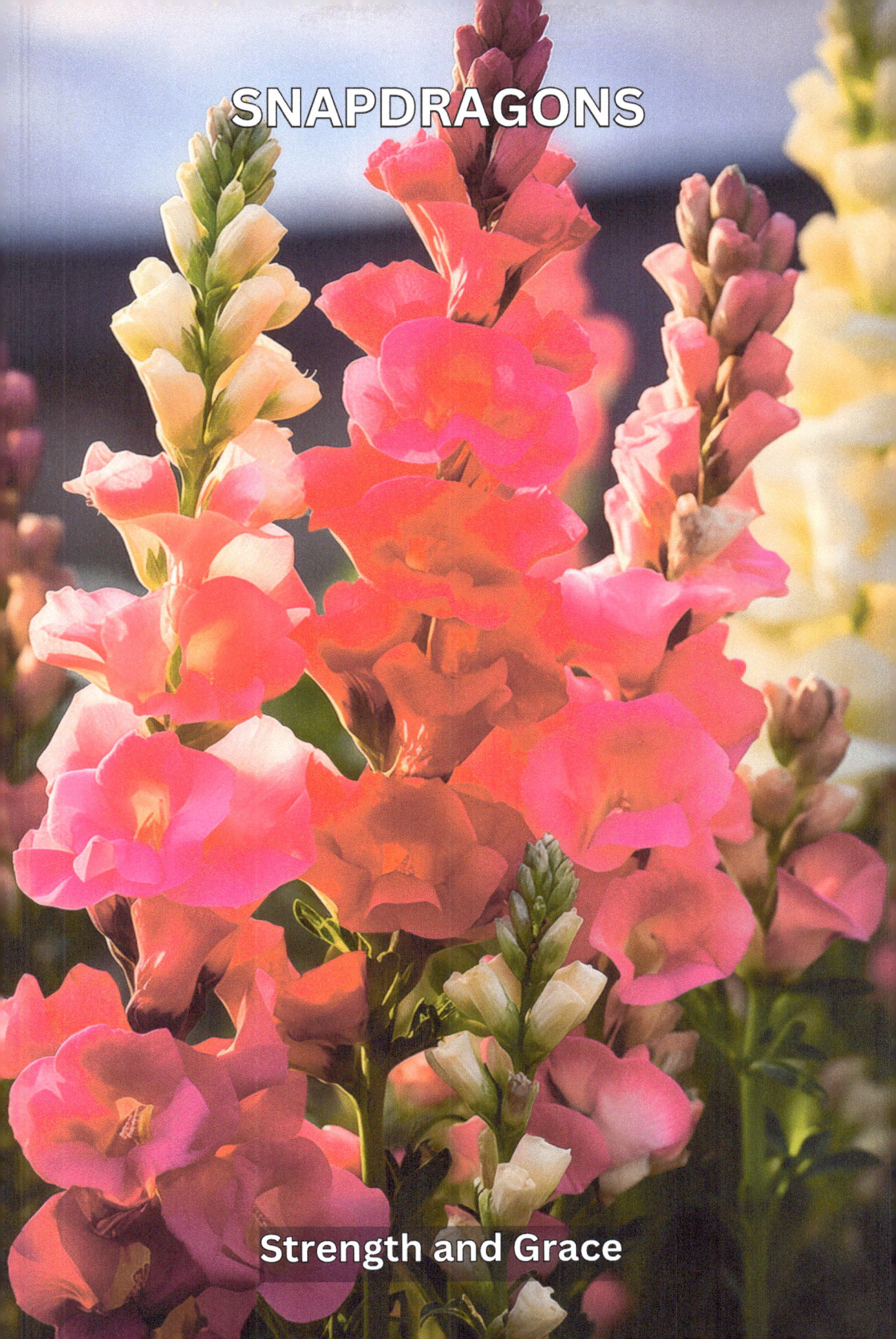

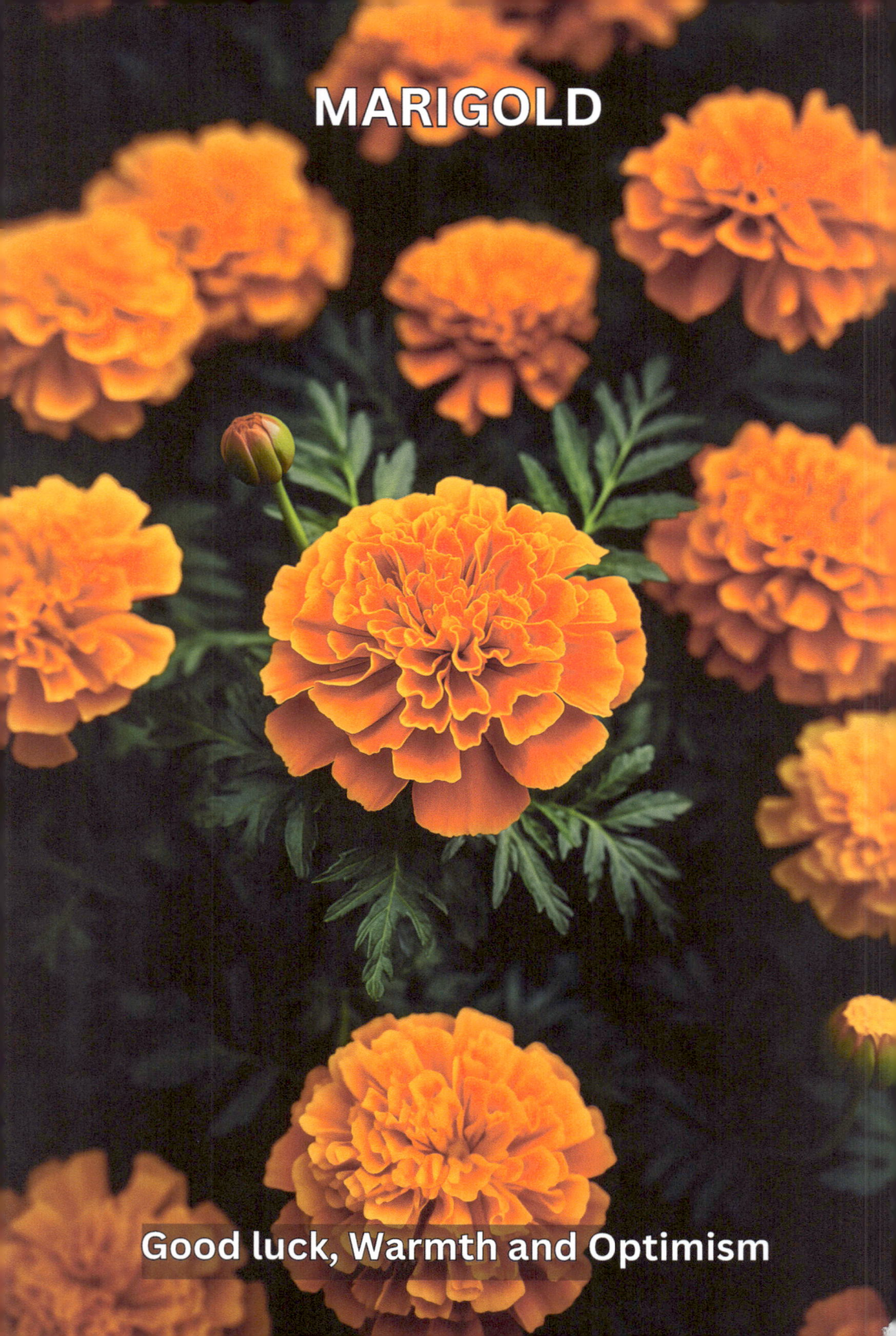

www.ingramcontent.com/pod-product-compliance
Lightning Source LLC
Chambersburg PA
CBHW040243220526
45473CB00001B/357